Another Cup

An Anthology of Encounters

VERA WATERS

Penn Cottage Books

ISBN 978-0-9516952-8-9

A catalogue record for this book is available from the British Library.

First published by Penn Cottage Books 2017

Penn Cottage Books, PO Box 121,
Chorley, Lancashire, PR6 8GF
Tel: 0845 838 7403

Printed and bound by Fretwell Print and Design, Healey Works, Goulbourne Street, Keighley, West Yorkshire

Cover Design by Heather Nelson, Photographer
nwheadshots.co.uk

For enquiries, talks & presentations:
www.verawaters.com

This book is dedicated
with love to my family

July 2017

Acknowledgements

Without the love and support of my family especially through difficult times this, my sixth book, would not have been possible.

I would also like to thank the following people.

Mike Gelder for his expertise in the world of high technology, also for his patience throughout.
www.redleg.net

Christine Blocksidge for her support and her dedicated help with the proofing & compilation.

Heather Nelson for photography and cover design.
nwheadshots.co.uk

David Moore for his comments and observations.

Jo Bell for first 'readings'.

Scott Lebin, Chicago, for his introduction.

Peter Kinson for his long term wisdom and support.

Andrew Thomson for his advice and good sense.

Michael White who ensures I reach my destinations safely.

And to Mick Clarkson who helps in so many practical ways.

Also my special thanks to the 'Longton groupies' who for years have magically appeared wherever I am speaking in the county and to other readers who have become familiar faces or correspondents.

I appreciate the support of my close friends especially Sue who throughout reminded me that at times we are all 'daring greatly in the arena!'

My humble thanks to all those whose life experiences are recorded here.

And last but by no means least, to you the all important reader.

Contents

Introduction   9

First Words   12

Lock the Doors!   16

The Awakening   21

Emotional Intelligence   30

Huddersfield Examiner   36

We Are All Kites   44

A Noise on the Stair   50

The Kitchen Candle   53

Good to be Alive!   57

The Summer House   63

The Shirt   73

Let the pieces fall   77

Black Lace and Earrings   82

Old age ain't for sissies   93

Did Curiosity Kill the Cat?   98

The Inner Spirit   102

Apple Pie Day   107

Mediocrity   112

What religion are you?   116

The Black Dog   120

Why Tarry with a Tassel?   127

Let us be Joyful   135

The Magic of 'Now'   139

The Learning Curve   145

Two Ears, One Mouth   151

There May Be Giants   156

Well I Never!   162

Love's Young Dream   166

I'll Have You Know…   174

Not a Prayer   180

Another Thought   182

Afterwords   187

Introduction

From the moment of our birth to the last moment we spend on this planet, we each travel on our own unique journey. Part of our journey consists of the serendipitous encounters with other people with whom we interact. Thus there is a constant merging of a person's journey with that of another.

Vera Waters' talent is her ability to extract insight from people and their stories. I know no one in my life who demonstrates this skill better than Vera as she shares her wisdom about the essence of such moments.

We first met well over a decade ago and together we have shared moments that have formed and changed my own life's journey. I have learned so much from Vera as she told me about the many episodes of her encounters with people and their challenges. It is her ability to make stories come alive with color, sounds, and dialogue that draws people to her lectures. Her talent is the ability to use such stories to extract a universal theme about a lesson learned. In this collection of her experiences all of these elements are evident.

I have anxiously awaited for her to compile a collection of her life experiences. Her sharing of these moments allows me to read, listen, and hear her voice as she makes each episode come alive. I know for her they represent the unwrapping of the most precious gift she can give: the love and compassion for those who need help.

Whether she lectures, shares her written ideas, or counsels clients, Vera's interactions demonstrate her empathy, insight, and love. More than anyone I have ever known, she has demonstrated an ability to help people discover their own solutions to survive life. She works like a maestro discovering images that take troubled people to important places and helps them recapture moments of truth. She uncovers important issues to help people discover their own strength.

Vera has never given up on her family, her friends, her clients, her worldwide audiences or anyone who has needed her. It is indeed an honor for me to introduce this collection of important moments in her lifetime journey tied to the stories of others.

I thank Vera for being willing to share some of her

personal journey with us. Her wisdom becomes clear as events are uncovered. These episodes have provided me with insights that will change my perspective on life and I am sure the reader of this book will be able to tie Vera's perceptions to one's own journey.

Scott R. Lebin, RFC, CWS
Geneva Illinois, U.S.A.

First Words

This really is an anthology; a collection of stories, reflections, and much more. Where possible, there are hints of when and where events took place, and I have full permission to pass stories on for you to share. Often when I speak in public, I'm asked if I will write again about the 'Emotional Bank' and grieving, and how to cope with loss. However, I hope that you will find yourself experiencing mixed emotions as you read; that you will laugh, and see how positive a sense of humour can be; how important it is to see the glass as half full, when everything is suggesting that it is half empty!

I do believe that we learn something from every event in our lives; and of course no one suggested that this, our present existence, should be totally happy. The cycle of life goes on long, after we are gone, the seasons will continue to follow each other, and the darkness of each night will eventually change into the dawn of a new day. As with all anthologies, this book is for reading at your leisure, sitting in your favourite place with yet another cup of tea! Be assured that as you read I am reaching out to you.

We all recall our experiences in different ways, and when I take you back in time, I ask some licence if, chronologically, there is a slight disparity. It is simply as I remember from years ago!

My view, when I'm asked what makes people feel contented, is that loving other people, getting involved with those around us, remembering the importance of acts of kindness, all of this helps us to feel happier in ourselves. Happy individuals are usually capable of facing crises that arise in their lives, they do not run away from problems, they seek solutions and in so doing retain some self belief and respect.

We are all unique.

You are a special human being, you may not be capable of changing the whole world, but you can bring about change for good in your own corner.

This life is not a dress rehearsal....believe me it's the real thing!

Seize the day!

Vera Waters
2017

Lock the Doors!

The traffic lights changed to red as I approached. There I was, sitting in my stationary car, on a very busy main road. It was dusk, my music was playing. 1972, yes, it was along time ago. I had recently been appointed to a senior position in the Health Service. The lights were still on STOP, the driver behind me tooted his horn. I looked in the rear view mirror. Some people are so impatient, I thought, 'Keep your hair on!' I mouthed to myself, 'I can't move until the lights actually change.' The impatient driver sounded his horn yet again.

Suddenly the back door of my car was pulled open, and a huge Alsatian dog jumped from the pavement onto my rear seats. It was closely followed by a man holding on to the other end of the dog's lead.

As the man slammed the door shut behind him he said in a loud voice 'Well, we haven't got all day. The lights are on green!' He followed this with 'Get your foot down, woman!'

I was so startled that I did just that. Looking frantically in my rear view mirror I could see the dog's head, and I noted that the traffic behind me was not moving.

'What do you want?' I asked the man as we sped along the A6.

Trying to gather my wits, I reminded myself that each day I worked with psychiatric patients. 'Put your work head on Vera' I thought.

The man replied with an expletive, closely followed with

'Oh, my God, I am so sorry!'

It was at this point that I stopped the car, and turning around, very hesitantly, came face to face not only with the very large dog, who looked far from friendly but also an extremely red faced man!

The man started to open the door of the car saying 'There's nothing to be afraid of please don't panic. I thought you were my wife!'

At this point a car, almost identical to mine, pulled up and parked behind us. A woman, risking life and limb, dived out of the driver's seat into the path of the oncoming traffic. Cars swerved to overtake her as she hurried onto the pavement towards my car.

The man, plus the dog, tried to leave my car, both at the same time - making their exit quite difficult. The woman, standing now on the pavement, grabbed hold of the man's sleeve, presumably in an attempt to get him out of the car. At this the dog growled, probably unsure as to what was happening to his master. The woman released her hold, and man and beast literally fell onto the pavement!

Very gingerly I got out of my car…there they stood, a man, and presumably, his wife and a dog, beside two cars that happened to be the same make, model and colour.

She turned to him 'You great lummock!' she said 'Go and get in the car. You've frightened this lady to death.' He raised his hand, rather tentatively, in my direction before doing as she suggested. Only then did she turn to me.

'I really am sorry. When we were at the lights I realized

he had mistaken your car for ours. I sounded my horn, but he didn't take any notice, and when the lights changed, my car stalled. Are you alright?'

I nodded, by then a bit lost for words. The incident had shaken me, causing numerous thoughts to fly through my brain, when her relative had jumped aboard complete with large canine!

'I am now' I replied.

'He will be feeling such a fool!'

It was then that I started to laugh, and so did she. I couldn't stop laughing.

She said 'I think you might be in shock after having a strange man and a huge animal take over your vehicle,'

It was then, as he saw us laughing, that her husband got out of their car and came back to join us, minus (I was glad to see) the dog.

To me he said 'Thanks for seeing the funny side, I didn't mean to scare you.'

At that time I was married; I couldn't wait to get home and tell my husband what had happened. I needed a reassuring hug and a cup of tea.

When I arrived home my husband was reading the paper but I mistakenly thought that, despite that, he was listening to me as I recounted my experience. I was sure he would empathise, understanding my feelings of panic when the man jumped into the back of my car.

'I could have been molested 'I wailed.

'He could have been anybody, a bad person, how was I to know?'

I waited expectantly, listening for his reassuring

comments. I expected that he would sympathise and then together we would laugh about the whole experience.

There was a long silence and then after what seemed an age he said.

'Did you say it was the same model of car, exactly the same colour? '

I nodded 'Exactly the same 'I replied

'I was really scared.'

He looked very thoughtful 'I wonder if they bought it at the same dealers as us?' and with that he returned to reading his paper.

I, his loving spouse stared at him for a few moments before going into the kitchen to make a very strong cup of tea. Our two matching mugs stood as usual beside the kettle…. However on this occasion I ignored his as I made myself a brew!

The Awakening

Once upon a time there was a woman,
Her name was Serena.
She did not like her name.
She asked her mother why she had chosen it.
'I wanted you to be peaceful and grow up into a happy person.'
Serena thought this was a ridiculous answer that proved her mother's outlook was quite limited.
Serena had never been a peaceful child and now she was not a happy adult.
But she was.......... Very successful.
She owned her own semi-detached house.
Drove a very expensive car provided by the company for whom she worked.
She supervised a team of people, mainly men.
She had her own marked space on the car park.
Because the company were pleased with her work she received a very generous quarterly bonus.
She agreed with her managers not to let her colleagues of a similar rank know exactly how much it was, she did not feel guilty agreeing to this as money was very important to her.
She enjoyed luxurious holidays abroad crossing the Atlantic and other oceans in great style.
A man tended her garden twice a week. She paid him the minimum wage as she believed he was not skilled.
A matronly lady cleaned her house each day and made occasional meals, however, as Serena paid her cash she

expected to pay her less than the minimum wage.

After all she was just a cleaner.

Despite all of this Serena was not a happy woman.

She knew that she should feel happy and became angry because she could not understand why she felt as she did, not only about people, but life itself.

She had just one friend, a childhood playmate.

The friend's name was Daisy.

They had remained friends despite the fact that they really had very little in common.

They met once a week and texted each other once a week. Serena insisted that this contact by phone was on a Wednesday evening at exactly 6 45 p.m.

Obviously they were not very close friends.

One day when they were together Serena asked Daisy if she was happy.

Daisy smiled 'Of course' she said.

Serena didn't know why but she felt angry hearing this reply. Why was it that Daisy, who was so ordinary and unconcerned about the fact that she did a job with no prospects of promotion, could smile and say she was happy?

Serena decided to concentrate on her work and think no more about being happy.

Ten people worked in Serena's team.

They did not dislike her, nor were they fond of her.

They all felt that she was an 'odd-bod'.

She was not a bad boss nor was she a particularly good boss. She seemed indifferent to what went on in other peoples lives, especially theirs!

They decided that she needed to maintain keeping her distance and only be involved regarding work matters.

Since her promotion to their department they had learned, via office gossip, that she had strong likes and dislikes.

The girl downstairs in the finance office told Natalie, one of the team, that Serena couldn't stand men with facial hair.

When he heard this, Luke, also on the team, stroked his beard thinking 'that's me for the "high jump".'

'She doesn't like pets' they heard from some one else, followed by 'don't think she's had a boyfriend since she started working here ten years ago.' This latter comment came from a woman who had joined the company on the same day as Serena.

They heard also that their boss had parents who lived about twenty miles away.

They did not know that Serena found the visits to see her parents difficult.

Serena's parents were not getting any younger.

She hoped that they would not grow old untidily.

She noted when, in restaurants, that some older people did not close their mouths when eating.

On viewing this she felt sick.

No, she thought, I will not allow my parents to grow old untidily.

No silly behaviour, as with dementia, although she had to admit that they seemed alright mentally at the moment.... proof of this being in the fact that her father still completed the Times crossword and rarely made a mistake.

She had checked his paper when alone in the room.

Yes, all his answers were correct.

Serena was very good at crosswords.

She very rarely if ever made a mistake.

Serena found most older people singularly unattractive.

Her parents would have to watch themselves and their behaviour, still there was a good residential home close by their house and they had the money!

Serena had no intention of looking after them, but she would help to get them into the home at the first sign of dementia or Alzheimer's disease.

She would do what was her rightful duty.

Nothing more. Nothing less.

A year passed, during which time she did not think about happiness.

It was not on her life agenda.

She had been busy with her work for the company.

Life, to her, was about being in control, working hard, and making sure that she was not distracted from that purpose.

She accepted the fact that she would never marry or fall in love with someone.

It would mean getting too involved with feelings and emotions.

She had no intention of allowing that to happen.

Time passed until one morning after she had briefed her team, Louise, the youngest of the group, asked if she could have a word in private.

This was very unusual, as none of the members of the team had the confidence to do this.

Serena invited her into her office.

'It's about Luke' said Louise 'and his son.'

I hope it's not a personal problem, after all, the Human Resource department should deal with that, Serena thought.

She sat upright behind her desk, rolling her expensive gold plated pen around in her fingers.

'What does the girl want that could not be raised at the briefing?'

It was a bright morning; the office was filled with light.

When the pen in her hand was at a certain angle, the sun shone on it, causing a reaction.

A darting sparkle appeared across the far wall facing the window.

Louise noticed the sparkle and, momentarily distracted, watched it dance.

Serena, somewhat annoyed followed the girl's gaze.

She too saw the sparkle as she moved the pen.

For no apparent reason, and without warning, to her own surprise, she just stared, almost transfixed.

She watched the small brightness as it responded to the movement of the pen in her fingers.

Some thing inside her,

Deep inside, stirred.

She felt distinctly odd.

'Isn't it lovely' Louise said.

The girl sounded excited.

Serena felt her response.

Thinking, I must stop this nonsense.

We need to get on.

She realized that Louise was now looking at her and had already begun to speak.

'Luke's son would love to see that' she said.

'His name is Aaron.'

'They both knew from before he was born that he was brain damaged, but Debbie, that's Luke's wife, she agreed …well, they both simply knew that they already loved him, he had started his journey preparing for the world.'

'They would not even consider termination.'

'You see, they knew they wanted that baby, no matter what!'

Serena opened her mouth to speak, but no words came.

For the first time in her life she was unable to do what she wanted.

Her logical head told her to mention H.R.; however she couldn't drag her gaze away from the dancing sparkle on the wall.

She felt odd inside, almost dizzy.

Still she rolled the pen around in her fingers and the sparkle continued to dance.

For some unknown reason she didn't want the dancing sparkle to disappear.

'What is wrong with me?' she thought.

'This must stop.'

But Serena couldn't stop.

She was mesmerised, not only by the sparkle, but by Louise's words!

She looked at Louise.

Serena wanted to know more about Aaron.

The image of Luke came into her head.

Should she call him into the office?

Should she have some one in to record the conversation?

One couldn't be too careful these days.

She, suddenly, sitting there, facing a younger woman had become aware of something different.

She couldn't name it.

She still felt odd as though there was something stirring deep down inside her.

In an effort to take control of herself once more,

She laid the golden pen on her leather tooled blotter,

The sparkle remained, as though fixed magically in stillness on the wall.

She realized that there were tears on her cheeks.

This is so ridiculous.

When she began to speak, the tears were in her throat as well.

Her voice was not her own, as she began

'Please tell me about Luke's son.'

'Well......Louise hesitated, speaking slowly 'we wondered if....

Oh they were right, I shouldn't be asking you.'

She stood up abruptly!

'Go on' said Serena surprised at the quiet tone of her own voice

'Do continue.'

'What is it you want to tell me?'

Louise resumed her seat. She looked relieved.

'We are trying to raise money for Aaron, so that he can go to America for some special treatment that will be of help.

Although Luke and Debbie are awake with him twenty four hours a day, this treatment would really help, not only him, as he would probably live longer, more comfortably, you know what I mean, but caring for him would be just a bit easier…it's not a cure, they know that, we all know, but it would help so much. We are doing all sorts of things to raise funds, people are so kind and Luke and Debbie are so grateful.

People have been very generous, it is not just about the money we raise, it's about how close we have all become, because of this little boy. We all feel so grateful for even the smallest bit of help.'

Serena looked at Louise, whose whole face was filled with……

Serena at first was not sure what it was…. she couldn't describe it. Then, she felt again that stirring inside, and in that moment, she realized she knew what was in the girl's face.

Louise's face was full of love.

Serena had very little experience of love.

Her parents had always loved her, but she had shut them out.

Any man who had been brave enough to love her, had been dispatched with alacrity.

All that nonsense was about emotion, and Serena didn't like people who showed emotion.

She thought they were weak.

After Louise left the office Serena picked up the pen once more.

The sun no longer shone outside the window.
It had suddenly become cloudy.
She sighed, thinking 'What was all that about?'
And then she saw it!
The darting sparkle.
Can't be. Not possible.
The sun is not shining.
The sky is overcast.
The sparkle continued to dance.
She dropped the pen onto her desk.
Once again she was transfixed.
She felt so odd. So out of control.
Suddenly the clouds parted.
Sunshine flooded the room once more.
The sparkle stopped dancing across the wall,
Remained still for a moment and then,
Serena picked up her pen once more.
The dancing light was as before, when Louise had spoken of Aaron.

****

Once upon a time there was a young boy named Aaron.
Aaron still needs twenty four hour care.
He and his family are happy.
Aaron loves to watch the sparkles that dart across his room.
They come because there is a large crystal drop that hangs in the window ready to catch the suns rays.
'Aunty' Serena gave Aaron this present when she met him for the very first time.
She is now godmother to Aaron's baby sister Eliza May.

28

Little Aaron laughs at the sparkles that dart across the wall of his bedroom as the sun shines through it

When his daddy Luke touches the string that holds the droplet it moves, and he knows then that the magic sparkles will dance even more.

What Aaron does not know is how grateful 'Aunty' Serena is to be part of their lives.

This gratitude extends to the other members of the team.

When Aaron laughs
Luke
Debbie
Eliza May
And
Aunty Serena laugh too!

Emotional Intelligence

An avid radio 'devotee', I rarely watch early morning T.V. However today was the exception, switching on in the middle of the news gave me an unexpected boost to start my day.

The head mistress of a small primary school had introduced a new regime to enable children to cope with everyday life at school. At first it was not obvious exactly what she was trying to achieve, then as the report continued, the picture became clearer.

Her aim was to help children to develop their own emotional intelligence. My heart warmed, I wanted to stand up and shout 'You have my support, God bless you!'

Constantly I exhort people to consider, and then review, their own Emotional Intelligence Quotient. Many of them have thought previously that this part of them was of little or no importance, or even worse, are unaware that such a part of themselves exists.

'Never heard of it' said the owner of a large successful company.

'Does it make money?' he joked.

My answer to this obviously derogatory response was 'Of course it isn't about money but being aware of your emotions. Building on that awareness will help you to lead a more fulfilling life! You gain confidence as a person and consequently you become better at whatever you do!'

At that point I looked into his eyes as I concluded with, 'And, as you so enjoy making money, you may even get better at doing that!'

At this he laughed.

We laughed together. But that, for him was the end of a conversation he was unwilling to value in any way.

When we feel more at peace with ourselves, those around us benefit from our interaction with them. Anxiety and strain is lessened in our daily lives. The spiritual aspect of life is paramount. We are all a combination of Mind, Body and Spirit. Some people have a belief in something much greater than themselves, a faith to follow, however. The awareness of our emotional intelligence is not about religion.

Many people who take the time to question. 'What, where, how, when' are becoming aware of the importance of their E.Q.

It felt so uplifting to hear that this headmistress wanted to help small children understand. No matter who we are, where we are, irrespective of our position in life, our E.Q. is important to our sense of well being. It links closely with our S.Q. which is of course our Spiritual Intelligence Quotient. However we need not get too technical here; in short it is about caring, understanding and empathy.

I watched as the on-screen reporter talked about the school, how new children, who are experiencing their first day wandering around, often afraid and feeling apprehensive, are assigned to an older child. This child 'carer' helps them through those early, often difficult days.

To help the scheme to work more quickly, there is a bench in the playground.

It is a friendship seat.

A child feeling lonely lost or afraid has only to sit down on the bench and wait, usually for a very brief moment. Soon an Empathy monitor will come over, ensuring that the lonely child is alone no longer. These monitoring children wear special Empathy hats to make them much more recognizable to other children. As if this were not enough each child in a class is given a day during which they are treated as a very special child; a child of importance. They are all asked about their interests and hobbies, in other words, they are valued and given confidence and reassurance.

How wonderful!

They can also admit to feeling afraid or apprehensive, knowing that they will be supported.

All of us need to feel wonderful at some time in our lives. A child comes into the world to be loved and cherished. For so many children this is not a fact, merely fiction. They do not feel that they are wonderful in any way. The experts tell us that this lack of self esteem passes down from one generation to the next. Many of us have seen evidence of this pattern, but it need not be so. Lack of self esteem does not necessarily go hand in hand with poverty or neglect. Some of the most wealthy people lack the inner peace that can create self esteem. They have the trappings of wealth without knowing how to cherish value and love themselves. Extreme wealth creates many barriers – attracting so-called friends who are not genuine.

We can change the pattern of our life. Lack of awareness need not always be passed down to the next generation.

Some people make strong decisions to ensure that their own children do not suffer as once they themselves did. They are to be applauded. On the other hand it is worth remembering that a small, toddling child, although unable to translate fully all that is said, is aware of intonation of speech and the facial expression of the parent.

Once, whilst waiting outside a primary school to collect two of my Grandchildren, I watched as a four year old boy rushed towards his young Mum. Proudly waving a rather questionable daub of paint on curled up paper.
'It's a tree', he said proudly.
His Mum stopped her conversation with another Mum briefly, very briefly; in fact only long enough to say to her son
'Not another one!'
Then turning to her companion she said
'These paintings he does, that's not painting
 Looks like he's tipped the paint straight onto the paper.'
With that she screwed the child's treasured masterpiece

into a ball and told it's creator to put it in the bin.

Hard to believe?

Not really, simply another glimpse of life without empathy. However I will never forget the look on the face of that particular mother's son as, dragging his little feet, he did as he was told and threw the paper away.

Such power!

Such control!

Such theft!

Yes it was theft! This mother stole a part of her small son's self esteem. A part that could never be replaced, because no matter how hard we try we cannot bring back even one minute from the past.

Imagine the outcry from this same woman, a decade later, as she bemoans to all and sundry, the fact that she simply doesn't know what her teenage son is up to......

why will this boy never confide in her?

Experts may suggest that this Mother is passing on her own experience from the past. If this is indeed the case, how sad for her that no one loves her enough to tell her how her little boy feels.

The friendship bench in the school is a brilliant idea enabling children to cope with their feelings.

Feelings of under confidence, apprehension.

Loneliness, even anxiety and fear.

Fear.

Were you ever so scared that you felt you wanted to become invisible?

Do you remember how that felt, were you once that

child?

Obviously the headmistress who instigated the appointment of the 'Empathy Monitors' knows all about the way small children feel. It is so important to remember that often children are not encouraged to feel good about them selves. Many have to find guidance and reassurance elsewhere. Surely it is no coincidence that most adults, when asked if they remember a teacher who once taught them, will eagerly recount an experience with a nasty teacher.

Sometimes this is followed by a smile or a knowing look as they recall with obvious respect, the good teacher who influenced their lives.

Empathy is part of our emotional intelligence. Becoming aware and in control of this intelligence is powerful and life enhancing.

Huddersfield Examiner I
Coping with the Grieving Process

Soundlessly she places the pink china cup on the saucer and momentarily closes her eyes.

'He's still here you know. I can feel him. He won't leave me, not after all these years anyway. He wouldn't know what to do without me. He just can't manage. I dress him every morning – I put his clothes out – just to make sure he looks right.'

Opening her eyes, she suddenly sees her own reality. He, the beloved, the valued other half of this most human of equations is dead, life gone from his old familiar body, he has quit this 'mortal coil', and having so gone, will not return. At least, not in this life, and not in his usual form.

This is a glimpse of death in later years. No less devastating, but because of age, expected.

But what do we make of death when, prematurely, a young life is snuffed out all too soon? Our dreams smashed and shattered while the experts write of all the stages of our grieving as though, by simply knowing, we can 'pull ourselves together' and dutifully comply.

So much is written nowadays about the grieving process. Through our somewhat meagre learning, we believe that we have knowledge and insight into this part of living that is death.

Naturally, that which is born must die. It is the order of things. The natural order. Why are so many of us afraid of death? Is it only those who believe in a higher being, a greater power, who have peaceful acceptance of a life to come?

The elderly lady sipping her tea from the pink china teacup will no doubt speak to her husband, her best friend, her helpmate, until she joins him.

What a wonderful way to cope with this end-of-life experience, to go on speaking, maintaining a long-established conversation.

She will manage her loss in her own way, just so long as she is allowed to, until someone else decides to manage this lady in her grief. This management can take many forms; usually actions without malice.

Close family members start to make what they consider to be helpful decisions: 'Dad, me and our Janet will come over and sort out me mam's things, all right?' Why is it ever 'all right'?

Their dad concurs. Why not? It's by far the easiest thing to do, and, after all, through his own grief, he, if he is a father at all, glimpses their grief and lets them have their way! Too saddened to argue. Too lost to disagree. It is he, not they, who, in the arid desert of the long-shared double bed nightly stretches out his toes, to touch the long familiar form – to find it gone,

What do we know of grief – unless this awful sense of loss is ours, in part. Is it not true that, often when the griever speaks, we say these now immortal words: 'I know exactly how you feel'? Surely this cannot be so, for if it were, would I see you scurry into a shop on seeing me approach, to purchase something that you really did not want to buy? Would you avoid the grieving me with such self-preserving tactics?

How can you know exactly how I feel? Let's face it, if you came even near in your attempt to empathise with me, you'd at least give me a chance to talk. Just in case I wanted to, and if I break down and cry, does it really matter all that much? Can I not expect that you, as my friend or neighbour, or simply as another human being, will help me to cope with my tears, and in so doing, give me proof that you are trying to understand my grief.

Is it that my suffering touches memories of your own? Or simply reminds you that you and yours continue with your living. You can breathe, relieved that, this time, death has passed you by, and chosen another.

Perhaps to prematurely clear away the belongings of the dead could be delayed, while the closest person who is left feels able to decide.

Let me take you on a short journey, back to that old lady sipping tea. The tea has little taste now, and has long since grown cold as friends and family come and go. She strokes the cup, and seeks its meagre warmth, and then, to bed. His pyjamas are there, on the bed. Just like him to finish fully dressed, she thinks. Prepared and ready now for bed herself, though she doubts that sleep will ever come. Beneath the duvet, she holds the precious garments close to her. She cries for her Bert, realising now that, yes, he has gone.

Maybe for weeks she'll hold his closeness next to her heart. Merely fabric – no – a pair of pyjamas bought on a sunny Saturday afternoon in the Co-op. A trip uptown. She remembers it now, and smiles between her tears. Too long spent tramping round the market; she had called him grumpy as they hurried home to tea. Grieving takes time; so much to remember; so long to forget.

There was a time when we could say that birth and death were both inevitable. But scientifically, we have made such progress that birth can be controlled in many ways – but death remains, as ever, our adversary, unless we make the decision to accept that it is part of our life's cycle.

This article was originally published in the
Huddersfield Examiner 1998

Huddersfield Examiner II
Foreigner looks at Huddersfield

They had good faces. Good Yorkshire faces. But then, why shouldn't they have good Yorkshire faces?

For this is the land of the White Rose, and here I sit, and watch the world go by, in Peter's of Huddersfield.

It would be hard to decide how old these two ladies are as they sit, sipping their coffee in the café. They talk of waiting for a bus in a nearby village, and describe meeting a tough-looking man with a huge haversack.

They are worried, very worried, because they say he was waiting for the bus with a small child who was better dressed than him. They tried to question him but, from what they said, he gave little response, only to say the child was staying with him.

'What could we do?' they asked, as round about us people jostle their way, with precariously balanced trays, to already packed tables.

What could we do? What can anyone do? This was the cry from the lady who appeared to be the elder of the two, although after twenty minutes in their company, I felt that they were both of indeterminate age.

Their eyes sparkled; they were animated in their speech. They were concerned about a stranger they had just met in their own village. They could describe him, from is dirty hair to his huge backpack.

At a nearby table there sat a lady in a fur hat. She, too, was I believe, of pensionable age. Her skin was clear, pink and white. She seemed almost totally without wrinkles. What is it about this Yorkshire air in Huddersfield which makes people look so much younger?

This lady talks to her female companion animatedly, and I hear from a friend that she formerly worked in this store, and is well known to many of the customers. She is a joy to watch, as she greets people coming into the café area.

As quickly as it filled with noise and people, this small area begins to empty, and suddenly, without warning, my friend and I are surrounded by empty tables.

Our erstwhile acquaintances have gone. Busy about their business. There is the proverbial lull before the storm. Suddenly, a queue forms – suddenly, because so many people come at once, and yet again, the tables are filled, and people jostle to find vacant seats.

For me, Huddersfield is full of life. It is a town that I liked from the first moment I visited. I have asked myself a dozen times if this is because it houses two of the best friends that I have ever known in my life, who give me so much love and kindness and support, that I marvel that they came into my life at all.

One of life's small miracles!

Although appearing to be quite cosmopolitan, the town has managed to retain an air of yesteryear.

No, it isn't old-fashioned; it is just that the people who have live many years in Huddersfield pass on their own particular Yorkshire charm, their straightforwardness, which somehow does not offend by being too blunt.

There are many smiling faces, and, in the main, an acceptance of those who have settled among them whose countries of origin are far away.

When I visit Huddersfield, it is the only time in the whole year that I travel by bus. You see, the bus stops outside my friend's house. It's much easier to leave the car, board the bus, pay the fare and have no worry about parking.

The return journey is just as easy and convenient. But what an experience. What a multi-cultured band we are, as we ride on the bus into town.

I remember on one journey, a middle-aged man, hearing me speak, declared quite loudly that there was a stranger in the midst, a foreigner, he said, from Lancashire. I smiled then, as I smile now, remembering his words – for the bus was full of people of every colour and creed, and I, from Lancashire, was labelled a foreigner. How everybody laughed!

It was so worthwhile, and made me realise that, with a large helping of good humour, we would find it easier to cope with life and its many facets.

In Huddersfield I have done things that I have never done anywhere else, from riding on the bus to catching the train to Leeds.

With my work, I travel all over the country, but small journeys are a new experience. I chose Huddersfield as my starting point.

The walls of my house in Lancashire are covered with a collection of plates. It wouldn't do to count how many came from this town.

Car boots, enjoyable Sunday mornings with my friends; the second-hand market on a Saturday. Oh, what treasures I have reaped. And, do you know, when I hear people talking about Huddersfield, if they are at all scathing, I find that I jump up to support a place in which I wasn't born, and in which I have never lived. It is a town that I like and whose company I enjoy.

And if I am to be 'a foreigner' on the bus in Huddersfield, I'll be enjoying every minute of it!

This article was originally published in the Huddersfield Examiner in 1998

We Are All Kites

The young man shook his head as he was offered yet another drink.

'No thanks.' His friend was insistent.

'Oh, for goodness sake have a drink, what's all this rubbish about you not drinking? We went to primary school together, we grew up together, I know that you drink.'

'Not tonight, not tonight.'

'What's so different about tonight?'

'Can't explain but I'm not drinking tonight.'

With that his host shrugged his shoulders saying,

'Well if that's the way you feel' wandered off.

Simon looked at the people, he knew many of them, and then there were others who were strangers. Usually with a drink in his hand he would have been walking across to the woman in the red dress at the other side of the room, but without the drink suddenly he felt strange. Would she ask him why he was drinking coke, would the answer be 'I'm driving' really suffice?

All this was too ridiculous for words and why on earth had he agreed to it. It had all begun that morning at 7.30 am to be precise. He had arrived at the usual time, promptly, rung the doorbell only to find that yet again it wasn't working properly. He knocked hard at the door. She was there smiling as ever, his coach, his life coach to be precise. This was his third visit. As always he had felt undecided as to whether he should continue. After the first session, he was sure that he would never return. When he met her for the second time he felt more focussed, but the sessions were challenging. In a way he was surprised at how challenged he felt, his thinking stretched and questioned in some way, he couldn't quite pin down. This very morning she had talked about being in control. He had laughingly responded with a detailed account of how controlled he was in his work situation.

'Ah' she had said 'how well controlled are you in your private life?'

'Well, I'm not out of control if that's what you're suggesting.'

Her voice was soft and yet he was sure that if she were to say 'Off with their heads' then that's exactly what would happen.

'I'll give you a small task, are you up to it?' she challenged.

'Anything' he had replied, and at that moment had no intentions of carrying out any task she might set him.

'I'd like you to be teetotal for the next 10 days.'

'What,' he said, 'no drink at all?'

'That's correct, not even a glass of wine with your meals.'

'But I always have wine with my meals, I always do, that's who I am.'

At this she was silent for a moment and then smiling said

'I don't think you came into the world guzzling wine. It would probably have been your mother's milk or the bottle made variety.'

It was at moments like this, especially when she smiled, that he made the decision inside his head to stop all this coaching nonsense and never come back to see her again. Now only hours later, here he was at his friend's party. Ben was a friend he had known for years. Whenever they met the drink flowed, he would arrive by cab and go home in the same way. Usually at this stage of the party he would be well away, chatting up any attractive woman, speaking his mind and when the feeling of warm euphoria overwhelmed him some kind friend would put him in a cab headed for home. He had broken the pattern. That would give him a foolproof excuse if anyone asked. If that was the case why hadn't he said that to Ben. He hadn't said it to Ben because he knew that Ben would immediately ask him why he had come in the car when usually he came by taxi.

All this was becoming far too complicated. The woman in the red dress glanced across at him, she smiled, she had a beautiful face, very attractive. Was she with anyone he wondered, feeling the 'chat up' line coming on. Standing next to her was a tall man in a dark suit looking very professional, but there was no bodily contact between them, no knowing intimate looks, so very soon he decided that she was alone, merely making small talk with the man.

Ben was circling the room yet again.

'You looking at Elaine?' he said.

'Yes, I am.'

'Well, she is available.'

And with that he wandered off once more. All evening Simon drank his coke and all evening he watched his friends drink more and more. He watched them as their speech became slurred, he observed them with great interest as they laughed too loudly, roared raucously at each others somewhat feeble jokes, stumbled and at one point even fell down on the floor. Soon it became apparent to him that they looked particularly foolish. The woman in the red dress had moved very little, she was still with the man in the dark suit, obviously they were together after all. He decided it was time he went home. Looking for his host he passed close to her. She said

'Leaving so early?'

'Heavy day tomorrow.'

'Sorry to see you go', she said.

He knew that, at this point, he should say something, he could, there was a welcoming look in her eyes, a look he had seen so many times before, a look that said 'I like you, would you like my telephone number?', but instead he simply called 'Goodnight' to Ben and made his way down to the street, unlocked the car and sat silently in the darkness for what seemed like an age. Eventually he drove home and enjoyed the best nights sleep he had for years.

His coach had said 'Ten days without a drink.' 'Not a problem' he had thought at the time. 'I don't have a drink problem, why should it make any difference?' He could hear her soft voice 'I will set you a task.'

Simon was my client, extremely successful, someone with high ideals, goals firmly set, the pathways to them extremely well established. He fully believed that he was in control of every aspect of his life. He never expected it to be difficult to stop drinking for 10 days. At the end of the fourth day he telephoned me.

'This is hard work' he said.

'Certainly is.'

'But I'm getting there, because it's so ridiculous if I have to come back and say I didn't manage it.'

Of course he did stop drinking for ten days and after that he asked me to set other tasks for him to help him understand more fully how self control affects our lives, how invaluable it can be.

Many of us feel that we are in control, often this is not the case.

A friend of mine is without a T.V. for a while as she re-vamps her apartment. 'I don't miss it at all. I have the radio, my music.' As her friend I have to add that she is a very successful busy woman with so much going on in her life, but when I ask a client if they will refrain from switching off the T.V. or Tablet for a couple of days they often look at me aghast.

'But I don't watch television at all. I am too busy', days later they tell me how hard it was not to press the switch, not to refrain from so simple an activity..

One man said he hadn't realised that the T.V. was always on in the background.

'I missed it. It was really hard to leave it switched off.'

It is all about control.

The title of this chapter 'We Are All Kites' provides yet another example of control. We can fly high into the sky of life, but once we lose control, like the kite no longer earthbound, we can soon find ourselves entangled in the branches of a tree, literally trapped, going nowhere at all. Knowing how to moderate our behaviour, how to say 'No' to ourselves maybe a hard lesson to learn but with this level of self awareness we can fly really high without mishap after all *'We are all Kites in the sky of life'*

A Noise on the Stair

I heard a noise.

I was not dreaming. True I had dozed off whilst relaxing in the bath, but now I could hear someone coming up the stairs.

Foot steps, very clumsy footsteps, noisy, heavy, like a man wearing clogs. I grabbed a towel and got out of the bath, covering myself as best I could, then I looked for something with which I could protect myself. No use picking up the sponge or a loofah…there was nothing at all. Then there was another shuffling that sounded as though there was more than one person outside the door. Dear God, please help me I prayed.

It was then that I heard the man, or men, walk noisily across the landing into the main bedroom…now was my chance to make my escape.

Gingerly I opened the bathroom door and was about to step out and run down the stairs, when, on looking down, I saw a pile of sheep droppings. It looked so out of place on the surface of my brand new, hundred percent wool carpet. From the door of the bedroom across the landing, the owner of the said dollop of sheep-poo began to baa loudly.

'Ruth' I said,

'How did you get into the house? You've frightened me half to death, and you've ruined my lovely new carpet!'

Our pet ewe was not listening as I bodily tried to get her to the top of the stairs, whilst at the same time trying to ensure that the bath towel did not fall to the floor. I failed miserably, I have to say, as four hooves, two bare feet, and a very woolly, large sheep became entangled with the falling towel, which was carried triumphantly off on the back of the ewe.

I ran into the bedroom, retrieved a dressing gown, threw it on, and raced down the stairs in hot pursuit of the now not so loveable pet, who, by this time, was in the lounge helping herself to a bunch of grapes in the fruit bowl.

'Ruth' I yelled.

'Get out of there…… go back outside, PLEASE!!!!'

I tried to shoo her out through the kitchen towards the back door, only to discover that her lamb, Eli, on finding his mother absent, had followed her scent, and had he not found something interesting in the kitchen, would have been up the stairs earlier.

At this point, with a sheep and a lamb in the kitchen, to say nothing of a very patient, yet huge, Labrador dog, I began to feel that I was on stage in a Whitehall farce!

The dog and the sheep were good friends, as were all the animals we had, and at this point, Bess, my faithful lab, bestirred herself, and appeared to suggest to Ruth that they should all be outside. Not before Eli had jumped from bench to table, knocking over a basket of new laid eggs patiently collected before the children had left for school.

The three of them walked sedately through the open bottom half of the kitchen door, as though butter would not melt in their mouths. With bucket and carpet cleaner in hand, I walked upstairs to repair the damage and, of course, a good vacuuming was needed to get rid of the dirt walked in and through the house.

Much later, as I stood, fully dressed, mug of hot tea in hand, looking out of the kitchen window, I asked myself 'Was it all worth it?' Before I left the house for work, I gazed across the smallholding and smiled, reminding myself how lucky we all were to be living this life, and that it was all because I have a daughter, who loves not only people but animals!

Later, much later, that night, when the children were long fast asleep and the moon was full up my husband said 'Must have been a treat for you this morning, having a late start, do you feel better for the rest?'

There's no answer to that, but I thought the experience could have given me a headache!

The Kitchen Candle

Strictly speaking, it's a tea light, one of those shallow little circles of wax in which the wick will burn for hours and hours. It's very important to me. So often visitors made welcome in my kitchen will notice the little flame. Good friends know why it's there, whilst other people glance at it then look away, only to find that the flickering image draws them back to look again.

Perhaps my love of candle flame is rooted deep in my soul, being raised by very Catholic parents. My experience goes back to my childhood. In times of deep thought and sorrow I wend my way into any church, whatever denomination, to light candles, and as I watch the flame, I think deeply of people I love and life in general.

It is because of this that I decided that I needed a 'kitchen candle'.

Somewhere in this world there are people suffering. Read, watch or listen to the news as daily conflict reigns, with terrifying consequence, in so many places.

It is as though we humans are unable to live peaceably with each other for any length or period of time. Almost daily, British troops die, or are wounded somewhere in the world to what end?

So I in my small way I light my candle for those passing souls, for the families left to grieve, for the children who will never see again their loving parent. My kitchen candle burns for those incarcerated, for those who cry out in pain. For the little ones who are dying of hunger, for their distraught mothers who can do nothing to help.

My candle burns for the homeless and the desperate who are without peace of mind and any form of comfort. For the children who sleep on the streets.

You may presume that I am religious, not I. Perish the thought. I am a pragmatist. The nature of my lifetime's work has made me so. I have seen so much evidence of man's inhumanity to man that I sometimes ask myself why I am still working long after retirement age.

The other night I went to a 'leaving do' - you know the sort, where people enjoy a good meal, excellent wine and, without warning, slide into that wonderful state of 'in vino veritas'.

'Why do you still work?' asked a woman in a loud voice. 'Surely you should have retired years ago?' As a non-drinker, I was not protected by inebriation from the harshness of her tone.

I did not recall her from earlier days, though assured later by others that I should remember her, if only for her tactless remarks.

'As long as through my work I can be of help I shall continue' I replied, and it was then, in that split second, surrounded by laughing, chatting, people sitting in that busy Italian restaurant, that an image came into my mind of my kitchen candle. In my head there were a few seconds of silence, as I thanked God for all that I have in my life.

Often, when we see people staring into space, we use the phrase 'you are miles away'. I certainly was, for at that moment I was in my own home. I was mindful of all the aspects of my present life for which I am so grateful.

On returning home, my faithful Labrador left her rumpled bed, and with old and tired eyes, greeted me. I put the kettle on to boil; the fingers of the kitchen clock had recently passed midnight, the magic hour. With mug of tea in hand, I lit my kitchen candle.

A leading journalist, Peter Stanford, once described me as 'One who floats above denomination.' I bless the day I met him, for he knew me in an instant for what I am!

Sitting there in the candle light, I thought of passing souls, of crying hearts, and said my usual simple prayer there in the flickering light.

'Dear God, please help us all, especially those who are afraid and weeping in these dark hours.'

All was still in my kitchen, the yellow dog lay with her head upon my feet, the tea was hot and sweet, the house warm. My bed awaited me, but I did not stir as the flame cast its spell around me; that spell that first captivated me when, as a child, I stood before the rows of candles at the foot of the statue of Our Lady. My eyes, like organ stops, watching the candlelight enhancing the blue of her plaster robe. Not for me even then standard prayers, just conversations with Him or His Mother, but I know that, as that tiny spiral of flame reaches upwards through the air, that if I think positively, and offer my words from within my soul, that something good will happen. My kitchen candle is my own private ritual and message to my God.

Why not light your candle? Perhaps you like scented candles alight around the house....good. Why not give one of them a specific purpose. Do I hear you saying that you don't go to church or believe in God? Light one anyway and thank something greater than yourself, for everything that is good in your life. While we still breathe we live ....and there is so much in this world for which to be thankful!

But again please don't get the impression that this is a deeply religious message. Not so. Flames flickered as soon as human beings learned to create fire. It's not about religion it's about hope, helping people to feel positive in their lives, and at the same time floating above denomination! Me, religious never!

Good to be Alive!

She unzipped her hand bag.

'This is really difficult', she said.

'I don't know where to begin,

What do you want me to say?

I don't know why I am here.'

She closed her handbag firmly, zipping it tightly shut.

As though, by doing so, she was making everything safe and secure.

'Would you like a cup of tea' I asked?

'Do you do refreshments here, downstairs?

Do you have a kitchen downstairs?

I suppose your secretary brings you tea....'

She rambled on.

Words, tumbling out of her mouth in quick, nervous succession until there was little sense or order in what she was saying.

I left her, as I went to arrange for two cups of tea and biscuits to be left outside the door to my consulting room.

When I returned, her handbag was, once again, unzipped wide open.

Its numerous contents were in full view, as I glanced towards her.

'Is your handbag full of junk, like this' she asked?

She closed the bag, not before I had noted several packets of medication, and lots of unopened tissues.

I heard the tea arrive outside the door, and once again felt grateful to have staff who knew how I worked.

The woman finally stopped talking as she drank from the

china cup, and even managed to eat a biscuit.

After a suitable pause, I asked her why she had come to see me.

No referral.

A private arrangement.

Was it her own choice, I wondered.

'It's all wrong' she said

'I'm not at the right stage.

I've never felt angry.

They say I should be at the angry stage now, and I'm not.

But I really loved her.

We lived together for the last six years, but I'm not angry.

Why should I be angry?

They say it's part of the grieving process.

I've read all about it.

I really loved my mum; she was the best mum in the world.

When I came back home to live, she would get up each day and tell me that, no matter what happened in life, we had to make each day a 'Good to be alive' day.

We have to make every day count.

We are lucky to be here.

We've only got one life!

That's what my mum said, every single day.

Honestly, she did, every day.

How can I feel angry, when everywhere I go in the house I feel that she is still there?

And it's a good feeling.

I cry for her.

And no, I'm not in denial!

I know she is dead!
I've cried buckets.
I've asked her to send me a sign that she is alright.
I'm slowly sorting her clothes, at my own pace.
Taking my time, just like she said I should.
We went through all of this, before she died.
But with what I've read in books and on the internet, I'm not doing it right, am I?
But we had a plan.
My mum and me, we had a plan.
She talked to me, telling me what I needed to do.
We had this long chat as soon as they said it was inoperable.
We both cried and hugged each other, and I took as much leave from work as I could.
What if I'm doing it all wrong?'

****

The internet provides us with limitless information.
A tool for learning.
For increasing our knowledge.
This easily acquired information, coupled with the fact there are so many books written about bereavement, can take us on a journey. We may begin to question ourselves.
However we need to be aware that every expert has an opinion of their own.
As each of us is a totally unique person,
We will react differently to our own life experiences.
When it comes to grieving for a loved one, no two people are alike.

There are very few common denominators.

We all grieve differently.

For instance, some people, whilst grieving, find it difficult to make positive decisions. That's because when we grieve for some one we love, all our feelings are in our heart, not our head. We may become forgetful, irritable, snappy, unable to listen or concentrate when others engage us in conversation.

That's why we need good advice in regard to the administrative duties we have to undertake when a death happens.

It's really not a time to make big decisions, such as putting the house up for sale.

It is far wiser to leave such a big decision until after a year has passed.

Getting rid of clothes and possessions within days of the death is often a decision made by other members of a family. Although possibly well meaning, the suggestion 'I'll help you sort her clothes' may tell you more about the speaker themselves. That person, whilst doing something practical, may find it easier to cope. Why not leave the loved one's belongings until later, when you can sit in peace and grieve. Try not to let people coerce you in any way.

Consider postponing decisions about your own everyday life that involve radical changes.

When we grieve, we need time to adjust. How much time this will take varies with each individual.

We should avoid haste, if we possibly can.

And most of all, despite the awful emotional pain you feel, do acknowledge that you are not being your logical self.

And when that friend, neighbour, acquaintance or a passing stranger says

'I know exactly how you feel',

Remember they don't!

Let the voice in your heart remind you that the speaker, whoever they are, definitely does not know exactly how *you* feel, simply because they know how they grieved after the death of a loved one. Every persons grieving is unique, we make our own personal journey. However help can come on that particular day when you feel so anxious and confused that you say out loud 'I think I'm going mad!' It can come from a friend or colleague who takes your hand and says

'I don't know exactly how you feel, but when it happened to me I thought that I was going out of my mind but that feeling eventually went away.'

Time doesn't necessarily take away the pain, however for many of us the burden of grieving gets lighter.... slowly.

Sometimes very slowly.

****

She unzipped her handbag.

Taking out her lipstick, she asked if I minded her applying it whilst she was with me.

'Don't want to go through reception looking like this.

I feel so much better, and I'll do what you suggest, and I'll stop spending so much time looking up how I should grieve.

Now I know we are all different, and that there is no right and wrong way, it's like a big weight has been lifted, and I want to come back for another session to let you know how I'm getting on.'

'You know', she continued 'my mum would have been pleased that I came. A friend of mine had been to see you last year. She gave me your card.'

'Perhaps your lovely mum had a hand in all of this.'

She smiled.

'I like the thought of that' she said.

'I won't bring this handbag next time.'

'You know, so often I spill everything that's in it onto the floor, because I forget I've left the zip undone.

I'm always fiddling with the zip!'

Replacing her lipstick in her handbag, she firmly closed the zip, whilst I made a mental note that when she came to see me again, I would explain how the memory can sometimes be affected during the grieving so much so that, because we immediately forget what we have last done, e.g. zipping up a bag, we appear to be off balance or clumsy!

The Summer House

Her apron was short, stiff and white; it looked as though it was made of paper. My mother explained that this was because it was heavily starched, as was the cap that the woman wore. The wearer of the uniform was tall, and I thought her rather grand, as she stood inside the entrance of the largest house I had ever seen. She was holding a large silver tray. I was attending a party. My very best friend, who sat next to me in class at the Montessori school we both attended was seven years old. A couple of days before, I had overheard my grandma discussing the coming party, with my mother and my aunt. 'He's a Banker, contacts in town earns a huge salary, no wonder they can live as they do.' I didn't quite know what to make of that, my father worked in the steel industry. He was a manager. I knew all about steel, but very little about banking, apart from the fact that my mother said that we must save; and my father said that, for every ten bob you earned, you should save at least a shilling. Until that afternoon, I had not known that my friend's family employed two maids, both of whom wore the uniform that I was looking at for the first time. They reminded me of the waitresses that served afternoon tea in Affleck & Brown's in town, although *their* uniforms were less starched!

As we approached the front door my mother told me that they also had a housekeeper, a butler and a cook, who made all the meals, and, as an afterthought, she added, and of course they don't drive that Rolls Royce themselves.

My friend Katie had never mentioned any of this to me. I thought she lived in a nice house just like me, but no, Katie was, it seemed, decidedly different. Once, whilst talking at school, I had explained to my friends that my father was studying at Night School in order to better himself. Again, I wasn't quite sure what that meant, but one day, Lucy, who was very hoity-toity explained, in a very grand voice, that my father was trying to get up in the world, which left me even more puzzled, because I never thought of him as being a climber, and he was quite tall to start with so why would he want to 'get up!' That day I was coming face to face with a maid for the first time. Of course I'd seen lots of maids and butlers in the black and white films. My mum took me to the cinema each week. She had been very sad when the theatres and cinemas were closed, as the war progressed, and delighted when they reopened, but meeting a Maid face to face, well, that was quite something. Looking up at the young woman's cap, I completely forgot the purpose of the tray she was holding in front of her. My mum had explained that I was to place my gift on the tray, just as all the other children were doing, forgetting her prior instruction I walked forward towards the sound of music that I could hear. Mum pulled me back.

'Put your present on the tray, Vera' she hissed.

I did as she said, and was rewarded by a dazzling smile from the young woman, who had cleverly lowered the tray to make it easier for me to reach. Her eyes were blue, very blue I remember thinking how pretty she looked.

I felt very concerned about the fact that I was not allowed

to give my present to Katie myself. Moving from the restraining grasp of my parent, I found myself in a large room with a shiny wooden floor. A few of my classmates had already arrived, having been relieved of their coats by yet another maid outside the front door. My mother's face was a picture. She felt that I had let her down again. 'Your coat' she mouthed. For some reason I was still wearing my light blue, home made summer jacket.

She was embarrassed, but a kindly looking gentleman in a black suit suddenly appeared and took my coat away. The Mums were then ushered into another room, to wait for the musical part of the celebration, when they would be invited to re-join the group in the main hall, refreshments having been provided separately for them.

At that moment I wished that I could be like Katie. She had everything, but still, as I thought about it, I knew that perhaps not, as she hadn't even been allowed to look at her own presents, let alone touch them. Moving over to where she stood I gave her a hug.

'You live in this big house? You never said.'

I liked Katie, she was lovely, always laughing, and full of fun. The Nuns at school were very nice to her. No matter what she did she never seemed to get into trouble. Only later did I understand exactly why. Again it was my grandma who explained to me.

'Her father is very rich' she said.

'I've explained that more than once he gives a great deal of money to that school they insist on sending you to', (*they* being my parents).

My grandmother was not given to suffering fools gladly,

especially when they were aged seven. Her expectation was that if she told you something, once was enough, and you should remember. Her abrupt responses to questions asked did not detract from the honesty of her answers. My maternal grandmother was a mine of information.

As we stood in the big room waiting for the party to begin, I began to understand what my grandma had meant. At that moment a Magician appeared. I felt a bit afraid of him, especially when he took an egg from behind my ear, and everybody clapped their hands. Time passed, and he played many tricks on us before we were led to a long table at one side of the room. Katie sat at the head and we, like adoring sycophants, sat down either side. The table was resplendent, covered with food. More food than I had ever seen before. Rationing was at its peak, and most of us present ate very frugally at home. Cakes, jellies, sandwiches of so many different kinds, I couldn't even imagine that so much food could be in one place at one time. What a lot of ration coupons must have been traded for this, I thought!

Katie's mother explained that, after we had eaten, we could play on the terrace and explore the park, then when we returned indoors, a musical concert would take place, by which time our respective mums would have eaten, and been introduced to Katie's mother.

None of us were very clear about what the music would involve, however, after we had finished eating, the man who had relieved me of my coat, wheeled in a huge birthday cake on a buffet trolley. We all sang Happy Birthday and our friend Katie blew out the candles.

We were informed that we would each take home a piece of the cake to enjoy at our leisure at home, and extra cake would be provided for our siblings, should we have any! Recalling that day I realize that it was like a military operation.

Next the beautiful French doors were opened up along one side of the room. The three doorways faced out onto the vast rolling green slopes of the garden. This wonderful expanse was referred to as 'the park'. Katie said it was too large to be a garden. We poured out into the warm afternoon air, to find outdoor activities, to one side, a seesaw, to the other swings, miniature croquet and a small court, not for playing tennis, but badminton. Everything designed to suit small children. It was all so unforgettable that even now all these years later, I am often transported back to that day, and that special space in time. A private park, acres of grass all owned by one family...like the queen, I thought!

The maids came onto the terrace to ensure that no child was feeling left out or lonely, and being young themselves, they laughed and danced around, singing Ring-a-Ring-a-Roses. Holding our hands, skipping, playing, pushing us when we chose to sit on the swings; it was all so wonderful.

Then came 'The Farmer's In His Den' game, followed by team games. There was so much to do; the afternoon was full of activity. It was as though the war had never taken place, that we youngsters had not only survived the horrors but that those experiences were far away from this idyllic place. The memories of gas masks, air raid shelters, sirens and planes flying in to bomb our city were temporarily erased. We were safe in a magic capsule of time. It wasn't quite like that really; I knew that my friend's father served in the war. In fact he was a high ranking Officer!

Katie's family had invited everyone from our small school. We were probably seventy in number, all gathered on this most unforgettable of days.

Always curious, I looked across the huge lawned areas surrounded by trees and shrubs and longed to explore. Herbaceous borders lined small paths that led between hedges into other parts of the garden.

Would there be a vegetable garden, I wondered, like the one we had at home. I had my own garden too where, as well as peas and cabbages, I was allowed to grow flowers. I loved gardening, tending my small plot, so I wandered off to explore to see what I could find. Perhaps a secret garden would be hidden somewhere, and I would be able to go through a door and find everything overgrown and mysterious.

It was then that I saw it, a wooden building, strange in shape. It had windows all the way round, each one with a colourful curtain tied back with bright ribbon.

Two steps led up to the door that was open. I climbed the steps and, looking inside, I could see an old worn leather sofa. There were lots of cushions, and a table stood to one side, with an upright chair. A vase was filled with fresh flowers and there was a stool. The whole place took my breath away.

Going inside, I sat down on the sofa. The voices of my classmates seemed far away as they played on, safely supervised by the young maids. Sitting there, I noticed that the leather on my seat had worn so thin that the stuffing fought its way out, to escape to the light. I knew what the stuffing was made of, as whenever I visited the house of my Great Aunt, I was told to sit on a particular chair. It was prickly and it chafed the back of my knees when I told my grandma that it hurt my legs, she said that was because it was filled with horse hair. When I saw the holes in the leather covered sofa, I moved away from them, and lay back against the big floppy cushions. They smelt so nice.

I loved the little house. I wasn't sure what shape it was. It wasn't square, it wasn't round, it was so interesting with all its little sides. The windows at the back were so close to the trees that it was possible to see the leaves clearly, in close-up; it felt as though I was in the tree itself, whilst those to the front of the building showed views of the green rolling landscape, acres of lawns, seeming to go on forever.

I didn't want to go home.

I wanted to be with Katie, having this lovely place to play in.

I wanted to stay forever.

I wanted to touch and stroke every surface. To smell and feel everything within this small dwelling. It was then I noticed an ashtray on a little shelf. Next to it was a pipe with a three pronged tool close by. I knew what that was for, as my dad had one, and I had watched him clean the bowl of his pipe so many times.

On seeing the pipe I became a little scared; a man came here. Obviously he owned the small house. Perhaps he would be cross that I had walked in and looked at his things without permission! I dismissed this thought and snuggled into the cushions and promptly fell asleep! My mother later told me that I must have slept for at least twenty minutes.

The next thing I knew was hearing people calling my name, and as I drowsily looked out through the doorway, I saw my mother and the maids walking towards the little house. They were calling 'Vera, Vera.'

I got up quickly and ran down the steps towards them. But as I ran I told myself that one day I would have a wooden house exactly the same shape as this one with lots of sides. It would be my safe haven. There would be no bombs, no sirens, no air raid shelters and everyone smiling when I gave them permission to visit!

Even at that early age I had begun to dream.

I dreamt of a world in which everybody was kind and cared about each other.

There would not be war or rationing. Little did I know that the sweets that would eventually become available to children would still be rationed for a further seven years, and that my dream, like so many dreams, would take time and effort to be realised!

As I write this chapter I am sitting in my small summerhouse. It is octagonal in shape with windows all the way round. I come here to write my books, it is so peaceful. Since that unforgettable childhood experience, I have been fascinated by octagons. Rarely will you find me using other geometric shapes, even in my patchwork octagons are my favourite.

When this summerhouse was erected in my small enclosed garden I questioned myself as to why I hadn't ordered one years before!

Previously, I had owned huts, sheds, greenhouses and other numerous, extremely useful outdoor buildings, in which I had crammed a couple of chairs plus a table, and yes, many relaxing hours had been spent in those places. But when I watched the erection of this hideaway I knew I had at last achieved this childhood dream.

That day, so long ago, sitting on the worn leather sofa I knew I had found a magic place, I recall how the maids laughed, seeing me come down the steps. One of them said 'I like this place too, although we're not really allowed inside, only to clean it, but it is beautiful.' She smiled down at me with those lovely blue eyes.

What a memory!

Now today as I sit, as I write; as I meditate in this small private place I am reminded how lucky I am to be here at all!

So often when we look at a problem we see it only from one angle. If it is our own problem or the problem of someone very close to us, it is easy to let our emotions influence our responses. Commonsense can fly out of the window, once our heart is part of the emotional equation. However we need to note that all too often, there are other sides to each situation. Maybe there are three people involved, as in a triangle, or four as in the corners of a square. However, we need to see the situation from as many angles as possible, like the many sides of the octagon.

Throughout our lives we are surrounded by symbols. They all have a meaning. This shape is one of *my* symbols and it all began in that summerhouse so long ago.

Every moment of our childhood, every experience as we grow.

Every feeling, every response, every joy, each and every moment, prior to the present, contributes, adds to, enhances, enriches and can influence the adult we have become, provided we see it in a positive light. If some of your experiences have been sad, cruel or hurtful those difficult parts of your life are, despite the pain, part of your apprenticeship for the life journey to follow.

Step from the past, embrace the present and live life to the full.

The memory of that first summer house is as clear today as if it was yesterday, in recalling my childhood experience I am reassured that life goes on despite everything!

The Shirt

I was longing for a cup of tea, it had poured with rain the whole time I had been in town. Now on my way back to the car park, I intended to stop at my favourite café. I loved the ambiance of the place with its 1940s theme. The staff wore authentic dresses, the women with turbans similar to the ones my mother and her sisters wore during my very early years.

There was always a friendly buzz about the place, with Vera Lynn singing in the background as tea was served in vintage mismatched china from those bygone years. My daughter and I visited often, enjoying not only the excellent food but the total experience.

As I opened the door, I could see that the place was packed. Oh dear; and then I noticed a lady sitting on her own at a table for two. Would she mind if I sat with her? When I asked, she half smiled, slowly, as though it was an effort, then said that she was almost finished anyway, and planned to leave soon.

The young girl behind the counter nodded and smiled at me, silently implying that she would be over to take my order soon.

I looked at my table companion. She was dressed smartly, wore just the right amount of make up, lovely hair, but it was her eyes that held my attention. She looked so sad, so lost, far away as though she was unaware of the chatter and bustle of her surroundings. During the course of my work, I have come to know that look well; many of my clients and friends have looked that way, usually as they try to live through, and make sense of their own experiences.

'A penny for them' I said taking off my wet coat and draping it over the back of my chair.

She turned and looked at me as she told me that they were worth much more than a penny, and then in the same breath she contradicted herself, by telling me that perhaps really, they were not even worth a penny!

'Are you a regular customer here?' I enquired. She replied 'My husband and I usually pop in for a brew on our way back to the car park, on a Friday, when the market is on.'

I wondered where the husband was today, but guessed that something had happened to him, hence the sadness I could sense.

'I'm sorry, I don't mean to intrude, but you look so sad, are you………..?' My voice trailed away.

'He died, my Frank. It was very sudden, heart attack, and he wasn't there any more, after thirty eight years; my Frank just wasn't there for me.'

'Do you have a family?'

'No. I couldn't have children. We just had each other, just me and my Frank.'

'Shall I order a fresh pot of tea?'

Whilst we were speaking, my toast had arrived; it lay uneaten on the plate. 'Your toast will be cold.'

'More important things in life than toast' I said.

My companion looked at me across the table.

'I like your jacket' she said. 'Well' I said 'it's really a shirt. Pure wool and several sizes too big for me I know, but I like it.'

'Is it a gent's shirt?'

'Yes.'

'I thought it was. My Frank had a shirt like that. We were on holiday in Scotland. I bought it for him in one of those home craft centres. It was his favourite.'

'I'm not surprised, this one keeps me warm when I am working on my computer, and believe it or not, this came from Scotland, too.'

By the time the second pot of tea arrived we were on first name terms, and neither of us seemed inclined to hurry out into the rain.

'Elaine, my name's Elaine.'

'I'm Vera.'

As it turned out, we were both originally from Manchester, and although age was not discussed, the similarities of our recollections served to denote our vintage!

We exchanged phone numbers and were finally about to leave. Having paid our respective bills, we prepared to part company. I turned up the collar of my woollen shirt. It was then that Elaine gasped and stared at me, the colour draining from her face; she looked suddenly quite ill.

'You're wearing my Frank's shirt, that's my Frank's shirt, where did you get it?'

I was speechless.

'I bought it at the charity shop on Market Street. I like to make fancy home accessories, and I often buy shirts simply for the material, especially if they are pure wool. I was going to make it into a cushion but then I tried it on and liked it. It felt warm and comfortable.'

The lady who owned the café came to enquire if we were both alright, and we decided to return to our seats as suddenly there seemed to be more to be said. We ordered a further pot of tea. I said 'Are you sure this is your husband's shirt?'

'It was when you turned the collar up; I saw the bright pink stain. You see, I accidently touched it with bleach, but the shirt wasn't ruined as the stain only showed when the underside of the collar was visible, so my Frank said "no harm done."'

'Do you want it back?' I asked.

'Do you always wear men's shirts?' This from Elaine.

'No I'm an author' I explained. 'Sometimes, even with the heating on I feel chilly, after hours of writing. Men's shirts are much easier to wear, and far more comfortable.'

'I write true stories and I'm working on my sixth book at the moment.'

Elaine looked better, the colour had returned to her cheeks.

'My Frank read a couple of books a week; he wouldn't consider a Kindle. "I like the smell and the feel of a good book" he would say. You know, Vera, I think he would be really pleased that his shirt was keeping an author warm!'

Later, as we parted company, both of us knew that this was the beginning of a friendship. When walking back to my car, I hoped Elaine felt just that little bit less lonely I decided I must honour Frank's memory and finish the chapter waiting on my computer screen!

'Let the pieces fall where they may'

Virginia Wolfe

Do you believe in God?
Do you need God in your life?
Is it essential for you to have a belief in something outside of yourself?

During my life I have met many people who have described themselves either as atheists or agnostics.
Nine times out of ten I have found these same people to be incredibly spiritual in their views and outlook, although when I, in the course of deeper conversation, have said this to them, they have often responded with horrified looks and vehement denials. When this has happened, I have merely smiled, and as Virginia Wolfe says, I have 'let the pieces fall where they may' and simply changed the course of our discussion, thus avoiding any conflict.

After the first Gulf War, I debriefed many soldiers on their return from active service. One day, whilst working with a particular man, he suddenly asked me if I believed in God. I responded initially by explaining that, as a counsellor, the content of our session should not include information about me, however it was obvious that he needed to know. I thought for a moment, and then I said 'Yes, I believe in a God and what I perceive him to be.'

Immediately he asked 'What is your God like?'

'He is a God of goodness, without anger or wrath, and he is not contained within any given religion' I said in answer to his question.

His eyes filled with tears as he began his story. He had been brought up in a very loving home where neither parent believed in God, or indeed the need for much restraint or control. As he continued to talk, I returned with him to his childhood, living in the country, playing with his friends out in the woods and fields all day, coming home for tea. He told me that his mother never complained if his clothes were dirty, as long as he was safely home and had behaved himself whilst playing.

'I had really good mates, we didn't get up to much mischief but we were certainly not angels.' He knew he was loved, he was never bullied at school, in fact you could say he had a very balanced and contented childhood.

His decision to join the army arose from the fact that his uncle, his father's brother, was a full time military man whom he hero worshipped from being a very small boy. Although life in the army was hard, he soon settled and was obviously very well liked. Popular with so many, he found himself becoming a 'confidante' to several other young men who, at their own admission, had led lives very dissimilar to his own. Whilst he had always been sure he was loved, there were others who had known little affection and respect during their formative years and beyond. Soon he began to appreciate how lucky he was in more ways than one.

He told me how his whole life changed when he went to war.

'Nothing prepared me, although I wouldn't want the army to know that. They did their best' he said.

For a while he was silent, perhaps he had talked enough for one day but no! Not so. We shared a brew and he talked on.

We were sitting in a comfortable room it was a mid afternoon that soon stretched itself into early dusk. I put on the desk lamp and closed out the increasingly cold evening.

'I don't like the dark' he said.

'Before this it never, ever, bothered me. Once, when I was a boy, a gang of us dared each other to walk through the church yard in the dark…me, I was the first through; a bit scared but not much! Now look at me.

My wife doesn't know what to do with a husband who wants to sleep with the light on!'

Suddenly he changed the course of our conversation saying 'If this God you believe in is really there, why does he let war happen in the first place? If He is so powerful, he could stop it all happening, but he doesn't, he does b…all!'

He swore in a non-offensive way, the words only serving to show how much he was feeling.

'Say something, Vera, please say something!' His request was full of anguish.

'Did you ask God to help you?' I asked him.

'Yes, I was desperate, I screamed at God but …..there was no God! Just like I'd always known was the case.'

This sorrowing, hurting man sobbed, holding his head in his hands. 'What use am I to my family now?'

The room was warm, not hot, just right in fact, but not for my client, who shivered with the inner coldness that deep emotional pain embeds within our very being.
I gently placed a blanket around his shoulders saying nothing. We sat together as he gently told me how he had watched his comrades die, the helplessness he felt knowing that he could not save a life, prevent a death or even ease their pain. The recollection that he had implored God to help him seemed to make him angry. He felt that this invisible God was laughing at the weakness he felt within himself. He had decided that this was a God of vengeance and wrath.

'How can anyone believe in a God who does nothing to save people?' he sobbed. We sat for hours….. he had so much to recall, to relive, to be angry about and most of it was directed at the God he was sure did not exist.

I met with him several times trying to help him to cope, to come to terms with his 'clarity recall' during which he experienced the most vivid flash backs. As the months passed we got to know each other well. Like so many soldiers he had to learn how to cope with the aftermath of war and the emotional scars that still cause problems, long after the physical wounds have healed.
For over a decade after our sessions ended he sent me Christmas cards, and then I moved house, changed my

consulting rooms, and although at that time, the internet was in its infancy, we simply lost touch.

When I think of him I have a lasting memory of our final conversation during which he asked me to describe not only 'my' God but to explain why I needed to believe in a greater being. As it seemed to matter so much to him I decided to answer his enquiry.

I explained that I needed God and a belief in the hereafter in order to help me through my life, that I found comfort in my daily conversations with this entity that I could not see. I explained that I did not pray I simply chatted to my God. At this he smiled, a special smile as if he understood.

Of all the Christmas cards he sent during the years he kept in touch with me not one showed a Robin or a sprig of holly. Not one snowflake or Christmas tree; they all without exception showed scenes of the nativity, the birth of the Christ child. Was that a thoughtful courtesy to me?

Did he ever eventually believe in the existence of God I do not know? As so often happens in my work I simply 'Let the pieces fall where they may' because, very often that is the wisest and kindest thing to do!

Black Lace and Earrings with Business in Mind!

We collided.

Accidently.

My fault.

I wasn't looking where I was going.

Luckily I was only small.

Six years old.

The frail looking lady with the dangling earrings and black dress understood immediately.

She held me firmly by the shoulders, pushing me back onto my heels, in order to see me better, as my mother began to admonish, me apologising for my lack of manners.

The lady smiled, an old smile even then, a smile full of kindness and love.

'Don't tell her off lass. She's only little. It wasn't her fault. I'm the adult. I wasn't taking notice either.'

My mother continued to glare.

'I said, it's not her fault!'

I loved her immediately, for there was no arguing with this black clad woman.

Even then I could tell that she was strong.

And with this knowledge came the hope that we would visit her often.

She was one of my mother's aunts.

Another of my great aunts I recall vaguely she lived in

the same area, in north Manchester. I went to her house once.

Just once.

Never wanting to return.

A visit not to be forgotten.

A litter of kittens, nesting in a bottom drawer beside the fire, their mother fiercely on guard, left a lasting impression on me.

Most unfriendly!

Even then I wasn't very keen on cats, and after contact with any feline, I came out in an itchy rash.

The cat-owning great aunt was, to my young mind, a person to be avoided if at all possible, whilst her constantly black clad sister was to be sought out as often as possible.

To me she was like a character read about in books stories written about interesting people, people who did wonderful things, like the film stars in the movies my parents took me to see each week at one of the five local cinemas.

I was an avid reader by my third birthday, and four years later I was subjected to read those dreaded Dickensian tales. Poverty ridden tragic stories usually about mistreated children so cruelly misunderstood! From then on I hated Dickens!

This woman with whom I had collided was very interesting I thought.

A character dressed differently to everyone else I knew.

Why the long flowing layered dress?
And her earrings with the beautiful ruby drops suspended on gold chains that reached almost the length of her long slender neck.
She wore her hair in coils around her head, white as snow.
Also when adults spoke of her they called her by name.
A strange name.
Sir Elin.

When I discovered why this was the case, I was middle aged, and she was long since under the proverbial sod!
But then as a small curious child, I thought it very odd indeed to call a lady Sir!
I ached to know more about her.
As time passed I discovered that she of the black dresses and long gold earrings was a force to be reckoned with, nothing soft was visible on the outside but beneath those layers of black lace and silk a warm and generous heart was beating
Stories of her activities spread quickly.
She was respected by most
Feared by some.
Loved by many.
And no one liked to be out of her favour.
She was a woman considered to have answers.
The gossips told of how her sons-in-law, at the end of each week, placed their wage packet upon her table, this was the order of the day, they were never heard to complain.
This was to ensure that all household bills were paid, and

children cared for, prior to the men assuming that they could call at the local on the way home from work.

God forbid!

As if they would dare!

From what I heard, the daughters made no complaint at this arrangement, as their mother did most of the worrying!

This pattern of home life on an estate of prefabricated houses was bound to be of amazing interesting for me, as it was the opposite of what I saw at home.

My parents strived so much and worked so hard to improve their status in life and consequently succeeded. We lived in a new build semi where I wanted for nothing, and went to a private school. Despite all of this I knew that my mum sometimes missed her relatives down town.

'You mustn't tell your dad we've been here' was always the instruction as we left after surreptitiously visiting them.

One evening in winter, we were sitting eating our evening meal when suddenly there was an urgent knocking at the back door.

'Edie, Edie called a woman's voice.

Dad answered the door.

My mum's second cousin Alice was clearly distressed.

She almost fell over the threshold, such was her anxiety and sense of urgency!

'You have to come' she said on seeing my mother,

'Me mam wants you. She's really ill. We've had to send

for Father O'Malley.
Doctor says she needs the "last rites".'
My dad gently but firmly sat her down in one of the fireside chairs.
'Did you know your aunt was so poorly?' he said looking at my mother, who replied that she had no notion.
'You need a brew before we set off' dad insisted, realizing the cousin had walked several miles and looked exhausted.
'No time',
'There's time enough, Alice' this said firmly.
'We'll both help, we will go back in my car and then if any errands need to be done, or anything fetched, I will have the car. It'll be much quicker. And our Vera can make all the brews, so the close family can stay close to your Mam.'
Alice gulped the tea whilst we three put on our coats.

In no time at all we were speeding down Oldham Road towards our destination, unaware of the scene that awaited us.
When we arrived, the whole of the extended family were filling Sir Elin's room. From there they spilled out into the tiny hall of the prefab, and into the front living room.
'Our Edie's 'ere'.
The word was passed from outside the open back door like a game of Chinese whispers!
'Let her through.'
'Let them through, our Alice is with 'er'.

Bodies parted to let us get closer to the great Aunt.

Bodies clad in navy overalls.

A man in a brown 'foreman's coat'.

A stranger in a suit like my dad.

A woman in a low cut, unseasonal dress that barely held her heaving bosoms in place.

Another woman wailing at the top of her voice.

My mother held my hand tightly as I was pulled through this sea of legs supporting straining bodies.

Then a mans voice, firm, not loud, but a no-nonsense voice, not to be argued with, spoke.

It was then I saw him.

The priest, by the side of the bed.

Complete with his white stole about his neck, he waved his arms in an instructive manner.

'For goodness sakes all of you, get out and let me do God's work!' he said in his very Irish brogue

Without so much as a murmur,

Some walking backwards,

Some stumbling,

Mumbling and whispering on their way,

All intent on obeying 'the voice of the Holy Mother Church.' Friends and family moved out of my great Aunt's room precisely as instructed.

I was too young to know why we were allowed to stay as the priest gave the 'patient' the sacrament of Extreme Unction.

At last, being able to stand at the foot of the bed, I was

amazed to discover that the receiver of this most reverent attention lay, eyes closed.

My lovely lady in black who always had a kind word was now

a wrinkled face upon the pillow.

Her breath laboured and shallow, as though every intake of air was a huge effort.

She was wearing what appeared to be a black lace bed jacket that ensured that no onlooker could tell if the nightie it concealed so well was white or indeed black!.

As the priest began to anoint the great aunt her eyelids fluttered momentarily. By the time he was finished we all heard a long sigh coming from the figure on the bed .

'Sir Elin' ventured the priest inclining his head in order to hear her last words,

'Is there something you want to say?'

Her tiny hands that had lain so gently clasped upon her breast, moved.

Clasped together no longer.

They suddenly waved in the air like two small birds released from captivity.

We stepped back from the woman who we believed was about to journey to join her maker.

The people who had left the room sensed that something had happened; once more they jostled for a place closer to the bedroom doorway straining to see Sir Elin take her last breath.

A voice was heard saying
'Did you see that?
Our Mam moved, she waved her hands.'
'Saying goodbye, perhaps' said another.

The priest tried again.
'My child, let yourself go gently into God's arms and all will be well.
Can you see the light child?'

Suddenly the eyes opened.
The breathing was no longer laboured.

'Father, will you please stop calling me 'child' and, no…
I can't see the light, and thanks to the Blessed Sacrament I feel a lot better!'

'It's a miracle!' someone in the doorway declared.
'The good Lord has saved Sir Elin!'
Well, I was very small, and in my mind I knew that I had witnessed…………just that. A miracle!!

People crowded around the bed and soon the priest was much restored to good humour after three glasses of port.
Sir Elin's daughters no longer wept
The several sons she had unofficially fostered over the years gave each other manly gladiatorial hugs.
As for my mum and Dad and me, it's my belief that we never found out what the great aunt wanted to say to us, and truth to tell, we were all so relieved that my parents

didn't, to my knowledge ever enquire further.

It is hard to remember exactly when Sir Elin died.

However it was a known fact that she received 'the last rites' on several occasions, always afterwards declaring 'The Blessed Sacrament has cured me once again.'

At which those members of her family who were present would agree.

'True, Mam, true. Will we take five bob up to Father for a Mass Offering?'

And always, the patient, port loving priest accepted the offering with incredible good grace. Telling himself that miracles occurred, especially on estates of prefabricated houses.

However because of these many and varied so-called miracles,

when she did 'pop her clogs', in true Mancunian fashion, the priest, thinking it was yet another false alarm, took his time in getting to the house, only arriving in the nick of time to assist with her eventual dispatch!

When I finally was told of her real name it was several decades later.

Because she had been the sister who took caring control of the family after her mother's death, her younger sisters referred to her as 'Our Sister Ellen' which then became 'Ser'ellen', which to my young ears sounded like Sir Elin !!!

When ever I start to write one of my stories, the characters come into my mind, easily remembered, because they left such an unforgettable impression on me, however coupled with that first notion, is my desire to pass on the lessons that I learned from what I experienced at that time.

Sir-Elin never gave up. I saw her as a strong person who dared to be different. Even when ill she argued with her maker as to when she felt it was her time to quit this mortal coil!
It is a fact, now recognized by the so called experts, that keeping active in body and mind promotes well being and good health. We live in an age where due to progress and scientific knowledge we are living longer.

In order to have an enjoyable autumn in your life the process of positive living needs to start in your spring.

I knew that Sir-Elin had always been positive, yes, she was controlling, with a big heart, a mighty strength, a distinct way of dressing that, as I recall, never changed, but most of all those with whom she came in contact accepted that, if she was on your side in any battle, there was not a lot to fear.

Even the strongest of people may need support at some time whilst on life's journey after all as 'pack animals' we are instinctively drawn to each other. It is a good idea to recall encounters with those people who have had a positive effect on our behaviour or our sense of well being, people we remember with a feeling of warmth and gratitude.

I am glad I met Sir-Elin I knew that she loved me although we were not frequent visitors to her home, but when I did meet with her, it was an unforgettable experience, one of the many that have influenced my thinking and outlook, I know that she made positive deposits into my emotional bank!

So often when the help of a counsellor is sought the client is seeking answers, needing support, comfort and guidance at a time when they are seeing the world 'through a glass darkly' As part of the therapeutic process I suggest that when visiting past memories they also embrace any recollection of a positive encounter no matter how long ago. These experiences often forgotten have definite healing qualities when re counted in the light of the present moment.

'Old age ain't for sissies…'

Bette Davies

Where am I?

Come to think of it who am I?

Some days I wake up and think, in those first moments, that I am young and vibrant.

And then I make my way to the bathroom.

At such an early hour I avoid looking at myself as I pass the mirror.

My reflection and I are not ready to parley in English or any other language - that conversation will take place later, when I am equipped to deal more ably with circumstances of my reality. After all, It was never my plan to grow old.

During my teens I passed through many stages. At fourteen, my father insisted that I should seriously think about becoming a nun. Returning from a three day retreat, I had made the mistake of declaring that I thought nuns did lead interesting lives. On hearing this he leapt upon the notion, almost before the words had left my mouth, and as a consequence, the number of silent retreats that I had been forced to attend - since the age of four - was dramatically increased over the next six months. Sadly, at least for my dedicated Catholic father, these disciplined events had the reverse effect he had hoped for instead of a agreeing to join holy orders I had made another decision.

I fell in love, in a literal sense, with Isadora Duncan, she of the scantily clad dances, who met her untimely death by wheel, spoke and scarf. Avidly, I read all that I could find, articles, references, descriptions of her life; and the photographs of her fascinated me. I became a follower and devotee. Of course my father did not know this. During what was to prove to be the last of the 'Retreat experiences', I told one of the most devout nuns that I had a 'crush' on the infamous Isadora.

As a result of this admission, my father was telephoned at his work, and instructed to come and collect his errant offspring. When his Ford car drew up outside the convent gates, the look of sheer shame and disappointment on his face spoke volumes, and the weeks that followed made me aware that - to my parents - I was a complete disappointment.

To escape from their obvious displeasure, I decided that I was not long for this earthly life, and that I would aim, whilst on this mortal coil, to become more spiritual, almost ethereal. Secretly I danced in lonely places, swirling scarves around myself, flinging off my stalwart shoes and listening to the birds as they chorused in the trees. So you see, I had no intention of growing old, as I believed that my existence would be done and dusted by the time I was thirty five... By then I would be a famous dancer who had just finished writing her autobiography, indeed, to add to the drama of my life, the last breath would leave my body as I wrote The End...very

Hollywood but then I was movie mad at that time!
Well it didn't happen …

Here I am totally unexpectedly, over seventy years of age.
Bette Davis was quite right 'Old age ain't for sissies', and as I type these words I agree with her wholeheartedly. However I have never forgotten Isadora I almost always wear scarves, my collection being many and various. In fact, I feel quite lost without one about my person, so Isadora will never be forgotten. And yes, I still dance every morning. Slower now, and that's the truth of it, but nevertheless it is part of my daily routine. I sweep and swirl, and in those precious moments when the music takes over my spirit, I am young again. By the time I speak with my reflected image I am washed and dressed. I then liaise with the mirror to put on my make up.

Every morning I awake wearing on my face the mask of Zorro, dark colouring down to the bridge of my nose and unless I want to frighten people, my concealer must be carefully applied and then, the magic of everlasting lipstick - (what a boon) - only when this ritual is complete am I ready to dance and welcome the day.
My professional life continues and so often I hear my voice make promises that my body will struggle to keep, but I live for the day, the time in which I stand and, I constantly encourage everyone else to do the same.
However, I am *not* growing old gracefully!
How on earth could I?

It is not within my nature.

Why is that you may ask?

I would reply,

Age is a number, merely a digit, a way of keeping records of how long we live but...

If we make a point of showing those close to us how much we love, value and respect them.

If we think positively, and try to keep ourselves fairly fit, eat good foods, and smile and laugh a lot,

If we nurture new and old relationships,

Try to treat others well

And most of all, listen more than we speak.

If we try to do all of these things we will age in a positive way.

No one enjoys being with a moaner some one who is always finding fault is not good company!

Don't let that moaner be YOU!

However if we value every moment, laugh when the obvious physical signs of ageing become apparent and remain grateful for what we can still achieve we can grow old with a strong spirit and in our mind we can be free as the proverbial bird! ....But none of it is easy and it 'ain't for sissies!!'

****

Isadora Duncan was born in 1877 in San Francisco.

She became a dancer, teaching in her mother's dancing school, not classically trained she preferred a more bohemian, free spirited style of movement. She was a feminist who wore flowing clothes and almost always completed her ensemble with a long scarf.

Her life was tragic. Her two young children were drowned in a car accident, whilst she, a few years later, was seriously injured in accidents involving cars.

In 1927 whilst driving her new, open top car, her long scarf became entangled in the hub of the rear wheel, resulting in her death. Her time on earth having been tragically cut short.

Did Curiosity Kill the Cat?

'Are you lonely?'

'I hear you're not married?'

'Did your husband die?'

'Have you got children?'

I felt as though I was being interrogated…but no, I was simply sitting in a bookshop signing my newest edition. What made it worse was that I was in one of my favourite places, a very welcoming book shop with helpful, caring staff.

I looked up into the speaker's face.

As I did so the owner of the shop came over to me asking if she could have a private word with me.

Surprised I assured the questioning lady and the people queuing behind her that I would be 'back in a minute.'

When we were safely out of earshot, the proprietor said 'I'm really sorry but I need to say that lady can be quite difficult, really rude, and sometimes very offensive. She comes here quite often, but she really unsettled the last author who came to do a signing. She buys lots of books, but is so sharp and rude to people.'

Thus warned, or shall we say, informed I returned to the table where the said lady and others waited.

As if there had been no gap whatsoever in the proceedings,

the lady took up where she had left off.

'Well, did your husband die?'

The people standing close to her gasped audibly

I looked up into her face

A woman in her fifties perhaps?

Grey eyes, pale skin and an unfriendly face, full of doubt, or was it simply curiosity?

She obviously wanted answers

How should I respond?

The way we react or respond in everyday situations affects not only our own well being but that of others.

I stood up, and as I did so, met the eyes of the now restless, slightly embarrassed people waiting patiently for me to sign my books.

'How kind of you to enquire about my private life, you obviously really care about me. Why not wait until I've spoken to these other lovely people and then we can speak together when I've finished?'

I smiled as I spoke. A man holding a copy of my book gave me a knowing look.

The shop owner, standing nearby, looked at me questionably.

I took the book being held by the person behind the grim faced woman., She, in her turn, smiled as I asked her how she wanted her purchase to be dedicated.

I resumed my seat.

The curious interrogator flounced off, turning at the door to say

'If that's your attitude…'

As she left the shop we all heaved a sigh of relief.

The man who had given me a knowing look said 'That was clever. No wonder you do what you do.'
The other copies of my book had been bought by people who it was a pleasure to meet
One woman said 'It's such a shame. She causes scenes everywhere. I dread seeing her on the street.'

Later, as the shop owner and I enjoyed a welcome cup of strong tea, we found ourselves discussing what had happened; mainly because she felt responsible. 'After all' she said 'it's my shop, and it wasn't nice for you.'
Although known in the local community, the questioning lady sounded to me as though she had little support, few friends, lived alone, and the shop owner said 'had never been the same since her husband left her.'
A couple of hours later I walked towards my car. As I left the shop I spotted the grey eyed woman walking towards me. I must say I wondered at that point how she would behave.
'Are you divorced?' she said, 'or did your husband die?'
Before I could respond, she continued 'Mine didn't die. He left me for another woman.'
We sat in my car for over an hour.

There was no quick cure for the bitterness she felt. An awful feeling that had taken her over completely: she was full of resentment. It was almost contagious as it flowed from her. She spoke quickly, words coming like bullets from a machine gun. No gaps, no pauses, just a relentless tirade.

'Even the children go to see him, rather than me.
I'm their mother! I just hate everyone. I can't bear to see people happy, especially if they are my age.'

Now I will not for a moment suggest here that talking to me changed that woman's behaviour. However, what I am saying is that we have no idea what really occurs in other people's lives.
Often we judge by what we see, and look no further, which in itself only proves how limited we really are.
What I will tell you is that we were in touch for quite a time.
No one needed to know, however although nothing was said, the owner of the book shop sent me a very plain 'Thank You' card. It was inappropriate for words to be spoken then, or indeed written, but now, years later, this story can be told. The bookshop closed years ago and my only wish is that everyone I met on that memorable day, if still in the world of the living, is at peace with themselves.

Did curiosity kill the cat?
Do we ask questions because we are curious?
Or do we ask questions because we seek help in the form of answers?

Curiosity Killed The Cat - being inquisitive about other people's affairs may get you into trouble.

The Inner Spirit

Fear is but a hand
that clutches at the heart
It draws the blood from every vein
and pulls the mind apart.
A sharpening of the senses,
an ice cold sweat of shame.
The feeling of failure and
need to take the blame.
Vera Waters

During the course of my work I have tried to help many people to come to terms with bad experiences in their lives. As we are all such unique and therefore different individuals, that help has taken many forms. Hurt in itself is debilitating, as is pain – especially emotional pain. Frightening, threatening or traumatic experiences can leave a mark deep within us. Physical injuries heal with time, but it is often much more difficult to feel healed within, deep inside.

This is Alan's story. I've changed his name - (despite the passage of years).

It was very dark, windy as well, and to cap it all, it began to rain. It was three a. m. on a Thursday morning.

I sat in the car waiting; would he come as we had arranged, or would he be so nervous that the effort would be all too much? Five minutes passed, ten and soon a quarter of an hour, perhaps I had miss-timed this next step for him.

'Oh dear God' I thought 'don't let that be the case.' It was almost a prayer.

And then I saw car lights coming towards me in the distance and soon his car was beside mine. We were parked together on the rough ground that led to the canal tow-path.

He got out and stood he looked taller than ever in the rain. Sensibly he had brought a large police issue torch.

'Sorry I'm late' he said as he opened my door. 'Almost lost my bottle. This is really hard.'

I linked my arm through his as we made our way across the sodden downtrodden grass towards the canal. It was dark and eerie.

'I won't ask if you are alright, Alan.'

'No I'm not, but I have to believe you when you say this could help me recover.'

'How long is it?'

'Fourteen weeks exactly, and I've never been here since, although it's where I used to walk the dog every day.'

'You'll need to tell me when we get there.'

'The exact spot?'

'Yes', I said, squeezing his arm, 'it has to be the same spot, the exact place where it happened.'

'What was the weather like that night, remind me Alan?'

I had not forgotten about the circumstances of that night; through our sessions Alan had told me every detail, but for him to find his confidence, I needed him to remember and remind himself. After all, that is why we were there, at such an unearthly hour, walking on the canal towpath, because, soon we would be at the place where Alan had been so viciously attacked.

This police officer with commendations for courage could not understand why this experience had affected him so badly. During one of our sessions he had said 'Physically I'm better; ten days in hospital and then back home, OK, a few scars still; sore to the touch. But why the fear? I've never been a coward even when I was bullied at school.'

Weeks previously, he had waited for me to give him an answer, I had remained silent until he said 'Please say something.'

Life would be so much easier if we had all the answers; I especially dislike those so called experts, some of whom are in caring professions, who have answers for everything. A bit trite I feel, for **who** could have all the answers… not a human being for sure.

Suddenly Alan stopped and pointed his torch ahead. The long beam of light illuminated the path for several yards……

'I can't go any nearer' he said.

We were there - or almost.

'Alan, we need to stand in that place. It's just a few yards away. Please trust me. Although I am so much smaller than you I have immense inner strength and I will look after you.' I looked up at him, saw the tears, and with all my strength and courage propelled him forward until we stood together in the very place where he had been stabbed in the darkness weeks before. It was here where his attackers had abruptly turned whilst being chased, and faced him. His baton was of little use against the three of them as they stabbed and kicked him.

Afterwards they fled, leaving him bleeding and battered, unable to move.

He lay on that towpath for what seemed an age,

Until his fellow officers got to him. He had lost a lot of blood, he almost died, and yet here we were standing together in the darkness in that place.

Miraculously, at that moment as we stood together, it stopped raining, there was a slight breeze.

He was still shaking but he no longer wept.

I bent down and picked up a small piece of stone from the ground and pressed it into his hand.

'Alan, what is today's date?'

'I can't think.'

I reminded him.

'Please Alan trust me; say the date - repeat it after me. This is the beginning of your future. This stone represents the pain you feel tonight.'

I closed his fingers around its rough edges.

'This is a new beginning, Alan. Let us throw away the memories of the past.'

Alan looked at me as I continued 'please throw the stone into the water.'

Imagine the scene - the two of us in the darkness; he - six foot, and me at five foot two standing there on the towpath at 3 a.m., torches in hand!

My dear man - as I recall, you were still shaking a little. I silently prayed as you raised your arm and flung the stone into the water; it went so far, such was your intent, that it seemed an age before we heard it drop into the water. I hoped that, with this act, you had taken hold of your courage once again, hopefully restoring your belief in yourself as a man.

As we walked back towards our cars there was a loving silence between us until you said 'Vera, why didn't you pick me up and bring me here in your car?'

Before I had time to answer you continued 'It had to be my own effort didn't it?'

This brave man retired from the service a couple of years ago, after 30 years; he went on to earn other awards for his courage and service and he pleased me greatly when a month after the night described here he sent me a photo of himself with his dog. I'm sure you know where he was walking…… yes, there they both were ……..on the tow-path! He had asked a fellow dog-walker to take the photo.

The human spirit can be indomitable, that is why when people seek to bully or control, it is our spirit they try to destroy. Sometimes we need help to keep our spirit intact. To rebuild our inner strength and fortitude, whatever form that help takes, it must always be wrapped in love no matter how strong the packaging may need to be.

Try to make your spirit strong, don't give way, work for your right to be at peace with yourself, and most of all, never lose heart. Without hope, we exist rather than live. Thank you Alan it was a privilege to be part of your story.

Apple Pie Day!

He was small and wiry, with tiny hands and feet. 'I am a Bantamweight' he would say, as he shadow boxed across the room.

'Your Granddad is very strong' – we were told as we watched him throwing mock punches at his invisible opponent. We loved him. His grey eyes held a twinkle whenever he looked at us. Our grandmother was very large.

'Your Grandma is not a big woman, she is big-boned' he would inform us, after we had received a severe 'ticking-off'. 'She has a heart of gold, and I love the bones of her!'

I believed that she loved him too, despite the fact that there seemed very little demonstrative affection between them.

He would sit on his Captains chair, beside the kitchen table and study the 'gee-gees'.

'Horses are beautiful, especially when they win races' he would say, grinning. Betting was illegal at that time, but a man known as Sam would take the bets to another man, whose name we never knew, to be placed. It was all very 'cloak-and-dagger', mysterious to us as children.

'Remember' Granddad would advise, 'bet each way. That way you may win less, but you have a better chance of winning something.

Grandma fed everyone who entered the house. Her visitors might well inform her that 'No' they didn't need a third helping of her delicious pie, but she elected not to hear them. The food she cooked was very tasty; we all loved whatever she managed magically to produce, despite the rationing restrictions.

She would give orders to her husband from the kitchen, her voice loud and distinctive. He would reply promptly 'Yes, Norah, I'm just doing that', or 'Just a minute, Pet.' One day I was spending the day with Grandma and Granddad. None of my cousins were there, just my grandparents and me.

Late morning found me and my Gran busy baking in the kitchen.

'Just popping out for my paper' Granddad said, as he put on his coat.

'Have you forgotten it's Voting Day?' said Grandma.

'No, lass, I'll go and vote while I am out.'

'I've already been; we need to get Labour into power.' She then talked about Workers Rights and employment. Granddad agreed with her before leaving the warmth of the kitchen.

The apple pies were cooked, and cooling. Lunch was still sitting in the oven, but there was no sign of the 'Bantam' Granddad. By mid-afternoon Grandma was very worried.

'He's a long time' she said. 'Go to the corner and see if you can see him, our Vera. He should have been back long ago.'

I waited on the corner; no sign of Granddad. Trying to be helpful, I walked up to the newspaper shop. Rose, the owner, welcomed me with a smile.

'Have you seen my Granddad?'

'Not since this morning, when he collected his paper. Come to think of it, I never saw him pass on his way home; Sam was asking after him, too, I think he had some winnings for him.'

I returned to my Grandma

She was sitting in the living room, arms folded, lips tight shut, hair standing on end. She looked very fierce!

'He's not there grandma' I said.'

'What do you mean, he's not there? Go up and ask Rose in the shop if she's seen him.'

'I did, Grandma. She's not seen him since this morning.'

By now it was five o'clock.

'Make us a brew, lass, and be careful, fill the kettle with the jug.' The majestic brass electric kettle dominated Grandma's spotless kitchen – it was enormous.

Dutifully, I did as I was told.

My mother arrived to take me home, took one look at her mother's face and whispered 'What's up?'

'What's up?' roared her mother. 'What's up? Your father's gone missing. We will have to find a Policeman. He could be lying dead somewhere.'

Taking a hanky from her pinny pocket, she started to cry.

'Let's think, Mam' said my mother.

'Make your mum a cup of tea.'

'Yes, Grandma.'

Later, we sat, tea in hand, the two women speculating on my granddad's fate.

No-one went to find a policeman.

It was then we heard a noise. Hard to describe it as singing exactly; nevertheless, the words of 'It's a Long Way to Tipperary' floated towards us on the night air.

My Grandmother's face stiffened, as did her now-folded arms, squashing her enormous bosom making it seem more huge than ever.

My lovely wiry, bantamweight shadow-boxing granddad was weaving his way along the garden path towards the front door.

"Ello, lovely lass' he said 'Are you waiting for me?'

Running back indoors ahead of him, I called 'Granddad's home. He's safe, Grandma.'

She stood to confront him. To me, as a child, he looked like a little Leprechaun. I wanted to save him from whatever might happen next.

'Norah! I've done it, my sweet. I've done something very naughty. Oh, and I've spent my winnings.'

'I can see that' she bellowed, making her way into the kitchen.

'No, Norah. More naughty than that' he giggled again, like a small child.

'I went to vote.'

'At least you managed that, before you got into this state!'

'Yes, but Norah but you will never guess what I did when I got there….' There was a long pause before he said

'I voted Conservative ha ha, not Labour' he began to shadow-box in a very wobbly way.

'You voted Labour Norah like you always do but I went my own way ha ha…' his laughter was uncontrollable.

No-one saw the missile until it was too late. It sailed through the air, above the kitchen table as though jet-propelled.
My mum grabbed her father, and they both ducked down, whilst I watched, amazed, from my safer position.
The pie seemed, like my granddad, to have a mind of its own. It went through the open kitchen door and smashed against the white papered wall of the hall.
Mum stood up, whilst Granddad's snores filled the room. He was fast asleep under the table.

'Home, now, Vera' my mum urged, pushing me out into the hall, where stewed apple and crispy pastry littered the floor.
'Night Mother'
'Night Dad'
'Night Grandma and Granddad.'
We hurried home.
As we opened the back door, my father called 'Is that you, Pet? Did you remember to vote?'

Mediocrity

'I'm really busy, trying to do so much, can't talk for long; you know how it is ....'

He then goes on to explain, in detail, exactly why he can't talk to me.

Why I must not detain him.

Take up his valuable time.

But the only person using up time is himself, and he doesn't even realize that he is wasting *my* time, and I might be just as busy as he believes himself to be!

I haven't had a chance to speak as yet.

Is he interested, I ask myself?

Is he actually interested in anything I have to say?

It's then that he says he can give me five minutes.

He has clarified the time by looking at his Rolex watch, and then he continues with an invitation to his office.

But as soon as he has ushered me through the doorway, he explains that I don't need to sit down, because he only has five minutes to meet with me.

Five minutes has already passed and as yet I've merely given him a nod of confirmation.

I have not said a word.

He has noticed nothing about me, my facial expression, the fact that as yet I've not spoken.

All that I did was move towards him on the corridor.

When I nodded, he presumed that this physical gesture indicated that I accepted how very busy he is.

Does my lack of conversation endorse his view of his

own importance?

I hope not, because that is not what I mean at all.

You see, I'm just observing him, as he stands there in his expensive suit, his recognizable aftershave, equally expensive.

And on his desk a veritable array of the most up to date electronic gadgetry now available in this wonderful modern age.

I wonder if he will leave a space between his words.

A small pause will do.

If he does, or when he does, I shall have to tell him, providing I can find my voice quickly before he starts speaking again, that I do not want to intrude into his busy, busy, busy agenda not now or ever.

I simply saw a well dressed young man coming towards me on the corridor.

And as I'd forgotten my watch and didn't really want the hassle of searching in my hand bag for my mobile, I thought I would ask him if he would tell me the correct time!!

****

During my first presentation in Chicago, I asked the members of the audience if they would think carefully about one of my own quotes.

'Spread yourself too thinly and you give everyone the gift of your own mediocrity.'

Although I've slightly fictionalized the described encounter, I'm sure we have all met people like this young man. They vary in appearance, build, and gender. Sadly they can be found in almost every walk of life.

I have met so many men and women who fit this description. They have such a great need to make sure that their value is recognized, that they must always appear to be busy; much, much busier than anyone else. However, this need is based on a great lack of confidence, and a need to impress.

It can also be related to a fear of being seen to be empathetic in any way. After all, a person continually on the move can hardly be expected to stop to help a fellow being! This is not to be confused with an agitated work pattern which can present as being dismissive, rather than efficient.

The best communicators are those people who speak to us for a few moments, during which we feel we are very important to them, and that they are listening to what we are saying. They are often good public speakers, whose aim is not only to keep the confidence of the audience, but to ensure that each of their listeners feels as though they were in a one-to-one conversation. The people with this gift ensure that everyone to whom they speak feels real, appreciated and fully acknowledged.

Whilst training public speakers, I suggest that they remember that their audience is full of the most interesting people, each with a story to tell. For varied reasons they have come to hear what the person standing in front of them has got to say.

Whatever the topic, if you are the human being who has the temerity to stand before a group of people, be they few or many in number, and in doing so believe that you have some wisdom to impart, then whoever you are, as Roosevelt said *you* are 'the man in the arena' and are 'daring greatly'!

Next time you speak to some one, help them to feel good about themselves. It may only be a chance encounter, but only you can give them the gift of your sincerity. No one benefits from mediocrity!

'What religion are you?'

I looked at the audience as they sat, row upon row, trying to work out who was making this enquiry. Having finished my hour-long presentation, I had then invited questions from members of the audience. The words were hardly out of my mouth before I heard the man's voice. As there were a lot of people present, and he – when I finally located him, was sitting close to the back of the room. I asked him if he would stand and repeat his question. He kindly did so however, before I could reply, he continued with 'and before you give us your answer, I'm an atheist, and I do not believe in any religion at all.' Some of the other members of the audience began to look uneasy, others commented quietly to each other, and a few looked agitated. This was not the way I wanted my talk to conclude. After all, this same large group of people had laughed with me, shed the odd tear, and hopefully, were to leave the venue experiencing some food for thought after an enjoyable experience.

I sat down on the chair next to the small table on the stage. I was wearing a lapel microphone, and everyone could still hear what I was about to say. All eyes turned to me as the questioner resumed his seat. This was my reply……………..

'During the early part of my career, I wrote regularly for The Catholic Herald. At that time, the editor was a well-known journalist and he did me a great service when he described me as 'floating above denomination'. Thanks to his correct description, I have been able to answer questions such as yours with this descriptive phrase. It is indeed how I see myself and my belief. However, do not be misled. My faith in God has rarely faltered, whilst my faith in my fellow man is sorely tried!'

The man who had asked the question leapt once more to his feet. 'God.' he shouted 'Tell us about God if you believe so much.'

Some members of the audience had swivelled round in their seats as the question was posed. They turned back to me for my reply. It reminded me of Wimbledon on a Summer afternoon, minus the strawberries and cream!

So, that night, I did just that……………………..

Yes, I told over one hundred people about my God, and what I perceive my God to be. It had not been my intention.

As a counsellor, I have always practiced self-discipline, never disclosing my politics or religious beliefs, or indeed details of my private life. After all, my clients need the time they spend with me to be all about them.

I spoke of the God of my childhood.

The God my father introduced to me at a very early age. I was born on a Sunday. People passing on the pavement, below the bedroom window, were making their way to nine o'clock Mass. Two weeks later, I was in that same Church being baptised. From then on, until I was nineteen, I attended, not only Mass, but every other Service. My father was what can only be described as an over-vigorous Catholic. At school, with the nuns, I was told so many strange stories about God that it occurred to me that he sounded as though he was constantly angry, always seeking revenge, and that every human being was full of sin. As a consequence, I decided that I didn't care for this God at all, and although, on a daily basis, I was lead to believe that I was personally responsible for murdering his only son, I, from a very early age, did not believe it, and therefore, in my own small heart, refused silently to take blame for this monstrous, barbaric act.

I felt that my very special God would be lovely.

The God I believe in, the God who has guided my life is surely

A God of goodness and mercy,

A God of forgiveness and understanding.

I trust him to see that I'm doing my best and that I am a Christian.

If I do, on rare occasions, feel the need to 'go to church', I am not at all fussy as regards denomination, hoping that, as places of worship are supposedly about goodness and godliness, that it doesn't really matter. However, sadly, having attended, I am often aware of the lack of either, as entering as a stranger to the flock, one is often met with suspicion and hostility. This is not so with the Society of Friends, otherwise known as Quakers, where for many years, I have found fulfilment in the welcoming warmth of the spiritual silence.

By the way, as far back as I can remember, I felt sorry for Jesus. Such a lovely man, who was tortured to death, but nothing could persuade me that I was responsible for all his suffering. Without my beliefs in his teachings, his example and his love of mankind – including me – I could not have lived my life as I have.

Some of us need to know that there is a power much greater than ourselves, far more clever and intelligent than anything that humans can create.

A power so immeasurable that, no matter how much we think that we know, or how cleverly informed we believe ourselves to be, we are but mortals, who must do what we believe to be right.

To love rather than hate. To treat others as we would want to be treated, and that to remember that, compared to this great power, we are quite small.

Having said all this, I paused before concluding…

'As I have spent time with you this evening, I know that, without my God it would not have been possible; but then, as the Quakers believe, "there is that of God in every man."'

As I finished speaking there was silence, not complete silence however, as quite distinctly, there could be heard the sound of some of my listeners weeping.

I asked … 'Any more questions?'

There was a movement near the back of the room. A man was hurriedly leaving.

'Ladies and Gentlemen' I said, 'Shall we all have a cup of strong tea and a biscuit – especially as that is the title of my new book, which I will be so pleased to sign for you tonight!'

Very few people hurried home. I signed dozens of books that night. On returning home, tired and spent, my adrenalin having deserted me, I stepped into the house. I filled the kettle, and as the water boiled, I sank into a chair and said 'Thanks, God! That was a close one!'

The Black Dog

Churchill spoke of having 'Black Dog' days. Years before he was born, other people, particularly writers and artists, talked of this experience. They mentioned the 'Black Dog', but what is it? You may have met the Black Dog; he may visit with you sometimes. Perhaps you become aware that he is there, particularly when the leaves fall from the trees and winter approaches.

What is the Black Dog? To what was the great man Winston referring? Robert Louis Stevenson wrote about the Black Dog, when describing a sullen person; as 'A Black Dog upon his back'.

The Black Dog comes into our lives at those times when we feel worthless, heavy, yet strangely empty. When we are affected deeply by everything around us, and nothing in our lives seems positive at all.

Many words are used to describe this condition, this malady, this malaise. If, as you read, you are wondering to what I am referring, then I can say 'Good for you; you must be one of those people who have never encountered the Black Dog!' Congratulations to you, you are most fortunate.

For those who do encounter this beast, it is important to have skills and strategies at your disposal, in order to ensure that you survive in a positive manner. Taming the Black Dog takes a great deal of common sense that needs to present itself in the form of a quiet determination to cope. When the 'Black Dog' makes an autumnal visit, we often call this 'Seasonal Affective Disorder'. When he prowls at other times of the year, he could have many names.

People who experience Black Dog days often describe them as times when they awaken, only to feel as though they lack lustre, and the glass of life at that particular moment appears to be 'half empty'. They feel pessimistic and to look on the bright side of life is too difficult, as they do not have the energy to be positive. Everything seems to be dull and lifeless, even the colours in our lives are not as bright. When in this state, we find it difficult to complete a task, and then, within moments, decide not to do it because it will take too much energy. We become disinterested in those we love who try to speak to us. It can be an effort even to listen, let alone comment.

If the 'Black Dog' gets a strong hold, you may not even want to get up in the morning, preferring to stay in bed and do nothing at all but waste the day.

Some people experience an increase in appetite, whilst for others, a missed mealtime goes completely unnoticed. Time loses its significance as night rolls into day. Our weight may increase or decrease.

Often, when living with the Black Dog, we decide to go to bed in the early hours of the morning. We don't feel tired, simply shattered and weary, but not sleepy. As a consequence, the following day, we stay in bed until dinner time. We have effectively turned our night into day.

Our sense of self worth suffers a setback, we lose confidence.

There is a strong possibility that we will cease to be

creative, especially if we favour the arts.

If we find ourselves experiencing this most difficult phase in our lives, we need to be aware of what is happening. Months later, when feeling better, decide that the next time the experience occurs, you will put up a stronger fight.

What can we do to help ourselves?

Consider the following.

Lift your head off the pillow and decide to get dressed. This may not be what you want to do, but force yourself.

Wear something bright in colour; no garish patterns or stripes, but something with a good colour.

Avoid black, navy, purple and other dark colours, after all, you are getting ready to face the new day, *your* new day!

Look in the mirror.
Yes, that really is you.

Try to smile, even if you only manage to grimace or scowl.

If you usually use make-up, this is the day to start wearing it again. Remember, your real vibrant self is simply hiding at this time.

Listen to your favourite music, or better still download

music that is soothing, bright or cheerful.

Remind yourself that you are still alive despite the way you are feeling.

Eat fresh fruit & vegetables in small portions.

When you put the food onto your plate, ensure that you can see a large part of the surface of the plate, in other words do not over-face yourself.

Little and often can be appropriate, rather than missing meal times, and then over grazing.

Are you up to date with your vitamins?

Have you had a general health check recently?

Find a pen and paper, and make a list of what you are going to do during the day. This list needs to include the simplest of tasks.

Tell yourself that the Black Dog finds it more difficult to hold on to a moving target! So try to keep busy.

Include on your list every small task, even the most mundane or domestic.

Then having done this, walk outside, whatever the weather.

If you have a garden, get out there, rain, shine or even snow. Experience a change of temperature.

If you do not have a garden, then walk a short way down the street outside your house. Breathe deeply.

Do I hear you saying that you don't want to meet with anyone?

I presume that you want to be in control of these feelings

you have….. so feel the pain and do it anyway.

Once back indoors, go back to your list. It is time to start your tasks and you have already achieved one of them. Congratulations!
The visiting Black Dog can cause us to be very self-centred. We lose all the capacity for empathy, because we are so busy thinking about ourselves. It is important to make sure that, somewhere on your list, is a task, or even two, that will benefit
someone else.

As you read this, you may be excused for presuming that the writer is one of those people who actually does not know how you feel when this condition becomes part of your life. Be reassured I have met this animal on many occasions, and as a consequence have learned the hard way to 'practice what I preach'.

Consider investing in a light-box. For many people this simple piece of apparatus really does work. Look at the various sizes advertised, and buy the largest that you can afford. Use it as you would any ordinary table lamp. If you feel the Black Dog approaching, use the light to thwart his arrival.
For a very common sense reason the 'Black Dog' does not like this piece of equipment.
Take a look around the place where you live.
Select your favourite chair, the one you identify as your own.

Begin to cherish yourself. Sit and rest, close your eyes. When you take a bath enjoy the bubbles, the scent. Try to breathe in the atmosphere.

Avoid watching violent or tragic films on the T.V. You may find it advantageous to avoid the news for a while.

If you feel that you want to weep, when you least expect to do so, forgive yourself. It is only the Black Dog biting hard! It will not last.

Drink water sometimes instead of your usual beverage.

Concentration can be difficult, and for some people, reading a book will be out of the question, however Magazine articles need a shorter span of attention.

Try not to judge yourself too harshly, remember you are fighting back. Explain to those you love that, although you are feeling low, you still love them very much, and that you want them to be aware that you are trying to cope positively with this very common malady.

Why not be like Churchill; give a nickname to this experience? Some people find that this helps them to feel more in control. Throughout this chapter I have used the term 'Black Dog' as he did. One of my clients called his experience the 'Green Parrot', followed by 'and I hate parrots!' Another 'Doom-days.' Another, a lady, called her visitations 'head–in-bucket' days.

So, you see, you are not alone, and by the way, you are *not* going mad. Remember, some of the most famous, clever, beautiful and talented people, so many of whom are involved in leading fulfilled and successful lives, also live with the Black Dog, and his occasional, and unwelcome visits. Perhaps it's the price paid for being gifted.

Disclaimer. *The author advises that it is extremely important that you see your doctor if this condition persists, as medication may be required to assist in your recovery.*

Why Tarry with a Tassel?

Tassel(n):
A tuft of loosely hanging threads or cords, knotted at one end and attached for decoration to soft furnishings, clothing, or other items.

I've ordered fifty.
Yes, fifty tassels chosen on a sunny afternoon in late May.
The year is 2016.
Why have I done such a thing?
Let's blame it on the internet, shall we?
Or the weather.
Or even the simple fact that I like tassels.
I always have, they fascinated me, from an early age.
My Grandmother, my mother's mother, was a wonderful seamstress, as indeed was her daughter, my mum.
Both of them made the clothes worn by the family, and every soft furnishing item needed for their homes.
One day my Grandmother decided to make a pair of curtains. The material was very beautiful, and heavy.
It was a deep rich, red colour.
First it rested as a huge, colourful mound on her lap, then, as she began to sew, it moved, slowly at first, then more quickly under the fast-moving needle of her sewing machine, across from her onto the table, from where it cascaded onto the floor.
It looked like an erupting volcano of red and gold.
It fascinated me as I watched its downward journey.

Because I was small, it seemed larger than life to me.

Its beauty took my breath away.

Soon first the curtain was finished.

Granddad was summoned from his vegetable plot.

He was, to give him his full title, James Francis.

His wife called to him in a loud voice.

Actually, more like a bellow, to be honest.

On hearing this, he knew that he was being commanded, not requested, to come into the house.

His assistance was required.

He was a small man. Wiry, bantam-weight, quick moving, agile, full of fun.

I loved my Granddad.

'Ladders!' said Grandma. 'I haven't got all day.'

The ladders were brought.

Soon, the first curtain was hanging in all its splendour from the big wooden rings on the rail.

'Looks lovely, Norah, really lovely.'

'I'll make you a brew, dad, and then you can go back into the garden until I've finished this other one.'

She pointed to the end of the long table where the remaining material lay, neatly folded.

Bulky, yet beautiful even in repose!

Before long, the second curtain was hung.

The effect was quite stunning, especially when the curtains were closed together.

All daylight was shut out.

When they were pulled open, they covered half the window at either side. The thickness of the material presented a problem.

Grandma stood back, giving herself a different view of her handiwork, and indeed the lack of full light.

'They need tying back!' she said.

We need big tassels to hold them back.

Deftly cutting into strips some of the left-over material, she shredded it, pulling the threads until they formed a fringe, which she then bound tightly, part way down.

These were attached to broader pieces that she tied around the curtains.

On completion, the curtains were positively controlled, letting in the daylight, whilst looking very luxuriant!

'And when they are shut, no light will show through; no problem with blackout' my Grandma said.

Because it was war-time, so much was unavailable.

There were many restrictions.

Clothing coupons.

Ration books.

And yet, it wasn't only Grandma that had the red curtains.

My house had them, too.

And my cousins' houses.

So many times, I have wondered where that amazing amount of colourful fabric came from.

My father had a saying, when asked a question he felt inappropriate.

'That's mine to know, and you to think about.' That was the answer I was given when I dared to enquire.

Throughout my career, I have gained quite a reputation for my work with people who were considered to be beyond help.

Indeed, once a friend told me of a comment she had overheard whilst at a social function.

The speaker was a smartly dressed man, who remarked in conversation

'That woman on St John's Street can sort out any problem.'

He was a High Court Judge.

'That woman' was me.

Some time later I met him and smiled to myself!

I have always believed that, when faced with a difficult situation we need to 'Think outside the Box.'

Every person is unique.

Totally unique.

Thank goodness.

We do not all fit in to prescribed pigeon-holes, no matter what the system, or the experts, would have us believe….

****

She did not speak.

My new client did not speak.

In her case notes, someone had written that she was……..

'Selectively mute and would need home visits.'

She did not speak to anyone.

Not one word.

I made my first visit to her home.

She lived with her parents.

Loving people, who wanted her to speak once more, but since she had been attacked, she refused to say a word.

Therefore it was difficult for the Police to discover and arrest the man who had hurt her.

Prior to our meeting several experts said she had decided to remain speechless because of the trauma.

As I looked at this sad, silent girl, I felt such empathy for her.

She was so traumatised, she had closed herself into a silent world.

There have been so many of these people in my life, classified by the system as 'selectively mute'.

Truly an apt diagnosis, as often they *have* made a decision based on fear and trauma.

Visit followed visit.

Welcomed by mum and dad, cup of tea offered, tears of anguish, and always the questions.......

'Is she getting better?'

'Will she recover?'

I could not reply in the affirmative. I could only suggest that they hope and pray, whilst I would do my very best to help their daughter.

One day as she sat quietly on her bed, I sang to her.

One day, I danced slowly around her bedroom, as she watched my every movement.

One day I played a tape of her favourite music.

One day I told funny stories.

That day, I saw the hint of a smile.

After my sixth visit, I began to feel that I had failed her, that even with all my experience and expertise, I could not open the door to her recovery.

At home one night, I'd tidied up after the evening meal, and I took out my sewing basket.

Patchwork fascinates me.

The joining of colourful scraps of material,
The hand stitching, peaceful, soothing and comforting.
I knew I would finish my project before bedtime.
I did!
The cushion was completed, the final touch being.....
A tassel attached to each corner, very pretty, gold strands
of brightness that hung from tiny, bright golden metal
caps, really too decorative for my patchwork, but they
were all that I had, and I was eager to finish this particular
project.

The next time I went to see the silent girl, I took a parcel.
It was wrapped in brightly-coloured paper, tied with lots
of colourful ribbons.
It was oblong in shape.
I placed it on the bed, and asked if she would open it.
'It's for you, especially for you. I hope you like it.'
We sat together in silence for the next fifteen minutes.
I remained totally still. The she put out a timid hand
towards the parcel – hesitating for what seemed an age,
she began to carefully untie the ribbons, which she then
laid flat on her pillows.
Next, the paper was removed.......
She looked at the cushion.
She smiled
A slow, hesitant, timid, facial movement.
She then picked up the patchwork cushion and held it
close.
Next, she put it on her lap, as she noted the details of the
fabric pieces.

Then

She began to examine each of the four tassels,

Slowly,

Carefully,

And then she said….. 'Goooollllddd, …..they…..are…..

gold…..

Vera…..they…..are…..gold.'

The words were elongated, as if each syllable gave her pain.

Silence followed until I said

'Do you want me to call your parents?'

She nodded. Gently I held her.

Mum and Dad entered the room, standing just inside the doorway.

She stood.

Held out the cushion.

Ran her fingers through the strands of one of the tassels.

'Goooooolllllllddddd' she said

'Gold'

'They are gold'………………

So many everyday things in my life bring back memories.

I know it can be the same for you.

We all have stories to tell, in fact, our lives are made up of our own true stories.

All are, as unique as we are.

We are all influenced by the lives we have led, and mine has been particularly fulfilling.

The young woman in this true account is as real as my grandparents, at the beginning of the chapter.

She did eventually recover, but charges were never brought against the person who had caused her to hide within her lonely silence. The last I heard, she had found love and motherhood herself.

The sun is shining, and a message on my 'phone from Amazon tells me that my order for the tassels has been accepted.

You know……………

I can't wait for them to arrive.

The corners of yet another cushion await!

Let us be Joyful

No one said that this life would be easy. Indeed many wise people have been at pains to make us aware how difficult life can actually be; and yet we meet individuals who always seem to look on the bright side of life, and it *is* possible for us to be like them.

Usually they are individuals who see the 'glass half full', unlike others who prefer to see the 'glass half empty'. When we meet some one who falls into the latter category, we have to ask ourselves do we really want to listen, as they tell us about how unfairly life has treated them. It can be a wise decision not to ask them how they are, as they might take the next half hour to actually tell us. One thing is certain we do not feel better for the conversation and often our own spirits drop and become sad and negative.

On the other hand the people who fit into the former category are often good to conversationalists; they leave us with a variety of good feelings, so much so that we may ask ourselves how can they be so joyful.

Joy can be found in the most unlikely circumstances, in situations that do not, from the outset, seem to be joyful at all. But life *is* unpredictable and it is the way in which we respond to challenging situations that influence, not only ourselves, but those around us.

During one of my presentations, a man suddenly began to wave his hand above his head like a child in school. It was a strong gesture. The man looked very angry; those sitting close to him began to move uneasily in their seats.

'Have you something that you want to say?' I asked.

'You, you' he said in a loud voice 'its alright for you, talking about joy and peace as though all of us can feel like that, you want to try being me. I have nothing to be joyful about!'

At that moment I was faced with a choice, the staff on duty at the venue began to move towards the man, fearing that his outburst might lead to something more serious. I glanced towards the steps leading from the stage on which I was standing, to the area where the audience were sitting. I walked to the top of the short flight of steps and stopped.

'I'm afraid I don't know your name.'

'Mark' replied the man.

'Mark, I'm wearing heels and I'm not sure I'll be steady coming to you down these steps, please would you give me a hand?'

There was complete silence in the room. The man stood up, then hesitated before edging his way in front of the other occupants of the row in which he was sitting. Eventually he was able to make his way towards me. Fortunately the two members of staff stopped and stood quite still. He made his way up the aisle.

As he walked towards me, I held out my hand, praying that he would extend his, and as he did so I smiled and thanked him.

He still looked angry and red faced, however he helped me down onto the main floor. Then I said 'Mark I owe you an apology, I did not mean to give the impression that feeling joy and happiness was easy.'

He then said, for all to hear, 'I've been out of work for two years, and now my mum has died, and I am not joyful, I am just so angry.'

It was as though we were alone in the room. I realized that he had forgotten that he was speaking in front of a large audience.

When he had finished, I looked at the people who had bought tickets to attend my presentation. Some of them were looking anxious and uneasy, others were straining to see what would happen next. A few were near to tears. The two members of staff walked back to their seats at the back of the hall. Still holding Mark's hand, I faced the audience.

'I know that we are to have a cup of tea at the end of my talk, whilst I'm signing my books, how about we all have one now? With that I nodded to the staff, they smiled, understanding what needed to be done. Off went the tea makers as Mark and I made our way towards the middle of the hall.

'We will all feel better after a cup of tea' I said, directing my words towards a lady with a friendly face. She took my lead and smiled.

Now you could say what was joyful about this particular experience. I'll tell you.

As we walked, several people smiled knowingly at Mark, some said they knew how he felt, One man reassured him by saying 'I think you need a pint mate, after all that…on me, when we finish.'

After we had enjoyed tea and biscuits, chatted and laughed together, the atmosphere became homely and relaxed. This lovely feeling enveloped us as we returned to our seats. Mark helped me regain my rightful place on stage and I continued with my talk.

As I prepared to sign my books, the people queued in a chatty, lively, warm line, having been assured by the staff that yet another cup of tea was on hand before they made their respective journeys home.

How absolutely wonderful!

Before people finally left (it seemed nobody wanted to go home), I said that one day, with their permission I would write about the evening and the huge amount of empathy and joy that we had experienced. Everyone seemed very pleased with this request, and promised to buy the book!

For several years, I kept in touch with Mark, and thanks to the man who took him for a pint, he did find work.

Mark, wherever you are now, I wish you joy, especially today as I write about that very special evening!

The Magic of 'Now'!

A knock at the door, my little dog barks, the doorbell rings, it chimes out noisily as I make my way towards the sound.

It's raining hard and yet the sun shines brightly filling the vestibule with brightness, whilst the falling water noisily assaults the windows. I open the door to find my young neighbour standing outside, his shirt soaked with rain, his girlfriend hovers beyond my front garden, equally as wet. My small dog Dolly, runs out barking, as if to say 'What's happening here?'

Phillip points upwards - 'I didn't want you to miss this' he says

'Have you seen the rainbow?'

Regardless of the rain, I rush out. A great sense of urgency assails me! A rainbow!! Looking up into the sky I see a full colourful arc stretching from the roof of my neighbour's house to its unknown destination. It seems to reach into forever.

A rainbow, a magical, mystifying, magnificent rainbow sent just for me!

You see that is how I feel about rainbows. They are my personal messages of inspiration and hope. I pray for these colourful curves to appear in the sky because I believe that rainbows are really special. Though not religious, I can empathise with Noah, sharing an understanding of his belief in what the rainbow meant. For him it symbolised hope.

The scientific explanations for this colourful phenomenon are proved and well researched but I choose not to lay much store by such scholarly findings, because I need my rainbows, and I have done so from early childhood. Maybe it was through listening to Noah's story that I began to look for rainbows whenever it rained. My parents told me that for a rainbow to appear the, sun had to be shining at the same time as the rain came down, but of course that is not quite correct as anyone who researches the rainbow will tell you - there are exceptions!. Their words gave me a rough guide and I became a seeker of rainbows and even to this day, decades later and a proud great grandmother, I have scars on my knees as proof of my diligent searching, for all too often, I fell over whilst running forward and looking at the sky simultaneously. One day I experienced a revelation. I was probably about five years old when, having fallen down, I saw a rainbow on the road in front of me. I was amazed, forgetting my skin scraped knee I looked closely at this mini arc of colour there, close to me, on the surface of the tarmac. As I watched it changed shape almost magically. 'A rainbow on the ground!' I declared to my father who was trying to assist with my now bleeding knee.

'No' said he, 'a patch of oil that has leaked from under a car.' This information led me on a learning curve, and from then on I increased my rainbow watch, ensuring that I looked up into the sky and not down onto the ground. However, now, when for a long period I have not seen a true rainbow, I am pleased to see the lovely imitations in oil slicks and reflected from hanging crystals!.

I hope that, on the day that I quit this 'mortal coil', a rainbow will appear…wishful thinking I know, but I can dream.

When in a difficult, sad or deeply worrying situation, when I have felt that I was unsure what to do, I have asked for a rainbow.

'Please send me a rainbow' I have implored 'please dear God send me a sign.' So often at those times my rainbow has appeared, not always I grant you, but very often. I've noticed that when people close to me die I often see a rainbow within the days that follow. Surely it is not all down to meteorological reckoning and occurrence, though my sceptics will insist that this is the case.

I am very fond of the southern Lakes countryside and spend quite a lot of time there enjoying the lush softness of the fields and valleys. One day whilst photographing a beautiful view beyond a farm gate, it suddenly started to rain heavily. As I turned to regain the shelter of my car, a rainbow appeared, quite suddenly, it was so beautiful I stood taking shots in the rain and felt renewed!

One of the nicest compliments I ever received was from a police officer who, being somewhat literary himself, produced a magazine. He asked if he could write about my work and, of course, my books. I eagerly awaited my copy of the publication. When it arrived by post, tore open the envelope, checked the contents then hurriedly found the page! His article was headed 'The Rainbow

Lady'. What a compliment. I was delighted and told him so.

A couple of months ago, whilst presenting with other authors at the Lancashire Book Fair, a tall man made his way through the crowd of interested readers. He looked familiar and yet I was not sure; in other words, as so often happens, I could not put a name to a face. And then his wonderful booming voice filled the room, as he said my name. It was Bob, who had so aptly entitled his article. With dark humour so prevalent within professions in which people cope with the horrors of life on our behalf, he said for all to hear 'Vera I will let everyone know that you're not dead, and as is only to be expected, you are still working' As I type these words there are tears in my eyes. A tangible proof of this deposit in my emotional bank.

Having spent so many years de-briefing professionals after traumatic events I have so many memories. Without my belief in rainbows I doubt that I could have continued for so long.

Elsewhere I have written about my time spent working with individuals and groups at the light station that I converted into a training centre in Scotland there it was possible to walk out early morning into the compound, and look over the white painted perimeter wall, across the wide expanse of the sea.

One morning as I looked out, a series of half and full rainbows appeared on the surface of the water. The sight was breath taking. I was so overwhelmed that I did not rush for my camera in case they faded as quickly as they had appeared. I could hardly speak. Then I heard one of the officers approaching. We stood together resting our heads on our arms leaning on the wall. Neither of us said a word. It was probably over five minutes before the rainbows began to disappear. They faded one by one as if reluctant to leave us. And we remained where we were in total silence for minutes afterwards, both too overwhelmed to speak!

Later that day the officer sought me out.

'I will never forget coming here for this training. It has changed my whole outlook on life. Would it be alright with you, if, one day, I brought my son back, here to see this place. I would like to do that and explain to him some of the work we have done.'

Of course I agreed.

We need to be mindful of every moment in our lives. To be aware of the moment in which we live. Rainbows help me to do this, and consequently, for me, they have a magic all their own.

Rainbows have always been seen as a symbol of hope.

Because of their beauty/colour there is nothing sinister about them.

Noah was the first person recorded as seeing a rainbow (Genesis 9).

God sent the rainbow as a promise to him.

For decades rainbows have been used to represent hope and reassurance.

They have been much favoured by groups to encourage

people to work towards equality and fair treatment

Children love to see rainbows, especially if they are given time to stand and look at them.

I use rainbows in some titles, not only because of their beauty and colour, but also to give my readers hope and inspiration.

The rainbow worked for Noah with his Ark, why not let the peace, hope and love in the rainbow influence your life. You only need to stop and absorb the message.

In Greek mythology, Iris is the goddess of the rainbow. She is said to travel on the rainbow whilst carrying messages from the gods to mortals.

The Learning Curve

The ward was spotless.

Immaculately clean.

Beds made with military precision.

The ward sister marched towards me,

A student nurse followed at her heels.

It was my first visit to this particular ward.

I had taken up my senior management post ten days previously.

The sister's uniform was spotless.

Immaculately clean.

She stood before me so straight and upright that I wanted to say

'At Ease, Sister'

I began to introduce myself.

'We all know who you are.'

My proffered hand was not accommodated by a welcoming halfway gesture, no handshake occurred.

'I suppose you want a tour of my ward?'

'If you have the time, Sister.'

'You are a visitor, I will have to make the time.'

The student nurse flushed, her face red.

'Thank you Sister.'

The tour was brief.

'Do you want to meet my patients?'

'Of course, Sister. After all, my department, hopefully with your co-operation of course, will be providing a service for the ladies.'

It was then I saw them...

The ladies.

Beautifully dressed.

Hair brushed.

All sitting at an angle, three sides of a square.

Some smiled.

Some looked vacant.

One lady appeared to be in a trance.

One lady was sitting knitting.

Bright red wool, that undulated in a wavy line across her skirt.

She was casting off, having completed a square.

I asked her name.

She opened her mouth, but the answer came from another orifice that did not belong to her.

'She's Nellie' said the Sister.

'Doesn't understand anything. Been here years.'

'How long?' I tentatively ventured.

'Ages, but that's not your concern. None of my ladies need to go on trips or meet volunteers. They are well cared for, and it's not as though they can appreciate anything.'

Nellie spoke at last as the final stitch of her knitted square was ready to by cut from the needle.

She held up the finished article gently waving the needle shoulder height.

'That's lovely' I said, 'really beautiful. We need to cut the wool. Are you making squares for a blanket?'

At this, the nursing sister whose ward I was visiting instructed the student nurse to leave us.

She gave her a task to do.

It was an urgent task, or so it seemed, after all it must have been urgent.

I didn't hear the words as these were whispered conspiratorially behind her hand.

The hand she placed in front of her mouth.

The young woman disappeared walking quickly.

Sister then turned to look at me.

A very piercing look.

I realized from the look of fear on the elderly knitters' face that I should be fearful too.

'We do not cut the wool, do we Nellie?' said sister.

Nellie looked down at her lap, and a tear was visible, venturing out from the edge of her eye.

'We don't need strangers to tell us what to do.' And with that, in one strong motion, she grabbed the wool, pulling the remaining stitch from the needle.

'This is what we do, isn't it, Nellie? We undo all of this square, row by row, and then Nellie rewinds the wool and begins all over again.

She knows it's for the best. We have no money to waste on wool!

Nellie, stop being stupid. Stop crying…..Now!'

The look on the elderly lady's face haunts me still. I'm probably older now than Nellie was then.

The matter did not end there, as you can imagine.

That evening I went home, and gathered all my spare, brightly coloured wool, and then, on my sewing machine, I fashioned a simple bag into which I placed the wool.

I found a brown luggage label upon which I wrote in big capital letters 'NELLIE'.

My appointment was that of a Senior Administrator, the first in the country. I knew the reason such a post was established was due to the fact that a huge inquiry had recently resulted in disclosures of large scale cruelty, and malpractice on the wards.

Patients subjected to the most awful abuse. My new post was set up as a safeguard to stop such cruelty ever happening again.

The next day I did not telephone the ward to let them know I was coming. I arrived with my bag of wool for Nellie.

Ignoring the worried looks of the nurses on duty, I walked purposefully towards the Sister's desk.

'Good morning, Sister.'

'You have no appointment, you can't…..simply … just arrive.'

The well-turned out Sister was so angry that the words fell from her mouth in disorderly fashion.

'Sister, I can go anywhere I want in this hospital. I have keys to all the wards. I am here to ensure that these lovely people, who are your patients, have links with the outside world.

Nellie, and any of the other ladies who want to knit, will never again be treated so badly.'

I lifted up the bag of wool saying 'This wool is for Nellie.'

'We keep them clean and fed, and they don't bother. They've no idea what's happening to them. Can't you see that?'

'Have you ever thought how the ladies feel when, having

completed a small piece of knitting, you unravel it in front of them? Don't you notice their tears?' I replied.

'I've worked here for years. The staff will have you out of here. We don't need people who know nothing of life on the wards telling us what to do.'

'Sister, I think not.'

Very soon the knitters made squares by the dozen. Staff helped them to attach the squares to each other, and then when the blankets were completed, they were donated to a local charity. What a wonderful time was experienced when representatives from the charity came onto the ward to meet the patients.

Prior to the enquiry, there were many staff who worked day and night in difficult situations, to provide care of a high standard.

I soon saw the good work. The level of care in so many parts of the hospital was exceptional, the standard of nursing excellent. The Sister I met that day genuinely felt that she was being professionally caring to a high degree. What was missing was empathy.

Fourteen years later, when I was leaving the Health Service, I was asked why I had decided to go, when I loved the patients so much....... this was my answer.

'The first time I stepped into this hospital a man was lying on the floor in the main corridor. He was licking the bottom of a radiator. Sadly sometimes he still returns to that same place on the corridor I'm leaving now before I forget the colour of his eyes!

Several people present asked my staff what I meant. Others, many of them nurses, nodded giving me eye contact across the crowded room. Progress and enlightenment had come too late for some of the totally institutionalised patients.

As for me I valued every moment spent with the people with whom I worked, both patients and staff, but I have never forgotten the look on Nellie's face, and how she looked on that first day when we met.

To make progress possible we need to change our outlook, our habits, our pre-convictions and our level of understanding. But most of all we need to accept that the whole of our life is a 'Learning Curve' of love!

Two Ears, One Mouth!

When she stepped forward, I could see the front of her leather sandals, and her thick white stockings. I wondered if she felt hot, especially wearing such a long flowing habit, and those huge wooden rosary beads. I wanted to ask her, but that was a very difficult thing to do, as I was small and only four and a half years of age. Looking back I recall that she was over six foot tall, but probably that is not quite correct as our memories can be deceptive. Could be that as I was small for my age, she simply looked enormous to me!

I had to walk with her, as she said her 'Office', round and round the quadrangle. My feet very soon felt heavy, and I was tired.

On seeing this she would stop and look down at me, put her finger to her lips and whisper 'Jesus suffered for us, we must do this for him.' She was never unkind. I liked her brown eyes and her face often smiled. If I was very weary, she left me sitting on a rustic bench, while she continued with her prayers; always when we finished she would say....'You have done well Veronica. Jesus will be pleased. One day you will be a very worthwhile person.'

I liked this nun, she taught me about perseverance, endurance but mostly about the beauty of silence.

By the time I was eight, I was expected to join in full day Retreats of prayer and silence. It was to prove to be one of the greatest lessons I was to learn. Often now, I remind people who read my books, or come to hear me speak, that it is not necessary to fill every waking moment with sound; that silence, as the saying goes, *is* golden, in that it has its own value, and is extremely useful as a form of self control.

I believe that, years later, when I spent time in the company of Quakers, I felt that I fitted in with their belief and practice of sitting in silence. Indeed, whenever I visit a Friends Meeting House, wherever it might be situated, I feel immediately at home in that gathering of silent prayer.

The ability to be 'still and quiet' comes through practice, and my personal belief is that, when faced with a confrontational situation, it's a good idea to be still and quiet, whilst you gauge what's really happening ; charging in with proverbial guns blazing usually achieves very little.

A fellow professional once said to me that this method of dealing with situations could easily be mistaken for lack of strength or courage; I explained that it takes much more willpower and courage to be silent and still! Needless to say, he had a loud voice and a rather more vigorous approach to life and its problems.

Once, when working with a small boy who, on several occasions, had packed a bag in preparation for leaving home, I was reminded how wise some children can be. What was he running from? It was my job to discover why he so wanted to leave home.

During the course of the time we spent together, he explained that he did not like noise. His parents argued and rowed every night, when he was in bed, he knew who was winning the argument taking place in the room beneath his bedroom, he believed it was the parent who shouted the loudest. He hated the noise of it all; he longed to be quiet when in his own bedroom.

Later when the parents were asked about their relationship, they were adamant that they never argued in front of their children

'We have friends who do that' said Mum 'We would never ever do it!'

Several sessions later, problems by then resolved, they admitted that they had never associated their difficulties within the marriage with their small son who packed a little bag in preparation for leaving home!

It's so easy to miscalculate how much a small child comprehends and notices in the adult behaviour that surrounds him in his environment.

Perhaps it's because of my early experiences in regard to silence that throughout my life I have needed to have periods of 'silent times' in which to be peaceful, to focus, to think and to contemplate.

However silence in a confrontational situation can be very powerful, mainly due to the fact that it is unexpected. It is different, and therefore varies from the 'usual' response, in other words, it often surprises people.

When we sit silently listening to what some one is saying, we give them permission to speak further, should they so wish. Often, in everyday conversation, people interrupt each other by finishing sentences, or by saying 'I know what you mean.' In doing this, we stop 'the flow' of speech. We cause the speaker to be distracted, or side-tracked.

One of the worst examples of poor communication is 'up-staging' or agreeing, using phrases such as

'That happened to me!'

'I'd have done that myself.'

Once we value silence, we learn to be quiet, to concentrate on what we are being told, at the same time acknowledging that our silence, our listening without comment, gives the speaker permission to impart their information in a safe confidential environment.

Throughout my career, I have trained many counsellors, however, often students would fail when asked to take part in a simple exercise, namely to refrain from saying 'I' when role-playing a client/counsellor situation. Of course, only the student taking the part of the counsellor was asked not to say 'I'. They fell like proverbial 'nine-pins', some declaring that surely it would help a client to know that the counsellor had had a similar experience. Not so. When a human being seeks help they seek empathy. If the counsellor talks of their own experience, they are reversing the roles. By so doing, they are demanding that the client empathize with them.

A good counsellor smiles quietly, when, at the close of a final session, the client says

'I feel as though you know just how I feel.'
Now that is empathy. Not achieved by saying too much! Away from the counselling situation, our interaction with those around us benefits from balanced conversation, one person speaks, one person listens, and we take turns to tell our stories to each other!

We have one mouth and two ears. Surely that suggests, even to the most garrulous of people, that we need to listen twice as much as we speak!

There May Be Giants

We are told of how Moses sent out his scouts to search for the land of 'milk and honey', a place where his people would be safe. A place to which he could lead them, away from the slavery they had experienced and endured.

When the scouts returned, they reported that, yes, they had found a land full of 'milk and honey', but that there were giants there, too. They had seen people who were very, very large and fearsome, the sight of these people had made them feel afraid.

A dictionary definition of a land of milk and honey describes 'a country where living conditions are good, and people have the opportunity to make money.' In other words, a place to be content and free. Moses was searching for somewhere that filled this description that would therefore be safe for his people to dwell. The report of the giants complicated things considerably. The scouts saw the giants as a major problem.

During my career I have met with people who, having found a good life, enjoy it for a while, and then become anxious, so anxious that they create their own 'giants' within the land of milk and honey, the good life that they have found.

Why does it happen?
This is the story of Jennie.

My receptionist telephoned to let me know that my next client was in the waiting room. Her voice was hushed and guarded.

'Could I come up now before you begin again. I have some papers for you to sign.'

'Certainly, the lady is early. Has she been offered a brew?'

'Yes' came the rather stilted reply.

My receptionist at that time, and I must say that during my long career there have been several, was a lovely young woman, married very happily, not given to moody outburst or behaviour considered unprofessional in any way. I thought she was a positive 'gem' so you can imagine how surprised I was when, having arrived in my office she presented me with a red, flustered appearance….not like her at all.

'There aren't any papers' she blurted out 'I just have to warn you. I know, in your work, you can cope with everything, but your next client is so rude and angry, mainly with me. I offered her a cup of tea, milk and one sugar, as she requested'…at this my receptionist became tearful, before managing to say eventually 'She sent it back twice. I've made three cups of tea. I'm sorry, but she's really got to me! She is so rude and angry!'

As you can imagine, a lot of TLC was needed for this lovely woman who was simply trying to be helpful, to assist me in caring for my clients. The care always began when the front door was opened. As a consequence, by the time my client was shown in by another receptionist, I hasten to say I was running at least ten minutes late.

The lady who had been waiting flounced into the room.
'What time do you call this. I've been waiting hours !'
'Do take a seat.'
Reluctantly she did so whilst saying 'I don't know why I've bothered to come in the first place.'
I sat quietly thinking of the paper file on my desk. It gave me little information, other than her personal details, and the fact that she was married to a senior consultant. Judging by the address, she had travelled over a hundred miles, possibly early that morning.
Looking straight into her blue eyes I said
'I have no wish to waste your time or indeed my own. Might I suggest that you either leave now, or refrain from acting in this angry fashion. You've obviously made a great effort to get here, let's not waste another moment, I continued without pausing. 'Did you have to get up very early today, or have you stayed in our lovely city overnight?'
She gasped, looked very surprised then replied
'I stayed at the Imperial last night. I arrived early evening and even went to a show.'
'Good. I've never stayed there myself, living locally as I do, but I often recommend it to clients who travel from a distance. I'm sure the service was as good as ever.''

The anger was gone now, pushed aside ever so gently, yet very firmly, by ordinary conversation that hopefully did not antagonise.
As this was a first consultation, I had allowed extra time. There was no rush. It was essential that she felt we had

time, time for her to reveal her giants!

In my environment she had been treated well, allowances made for the fact that often so many of us are anxious, when we seek help for a problem we are experiencing, whatever form that problem takes.

The 'White Coat syndrome' suffered by patients when visiting hospitals and clinics is well documented. It is a real fear. However there are other types of fear when seeking help for what appears to be a none physical problem.

Fear of looking foolish, fear of being judged, fear of being seen as a failure. It is because of this that so many professionals even in this more enlightened society still decide *not* to seek help.

One of my clients, a paediatrician, made a four hundred mile round trip to each of his sessions, whilst senior police officers also often made very long journeys to seek my help.

My team always behaved well, and I look back on their care of my clients and myself with great fondness and gratitude.

Every effort was always made to help combat these anxieties and to fully appreciate how emotional some people might feel.

As we progressed Jennie, (not her real name), told me of her fears. Her husband was well known, a prominent specialist in his own field, he was loving and generous in every way. However I was told he could be very grumpy after difficult days in the operating theatre. She wanted him to behave differently and felt resentful when he was too tired to be affectionate.

She told me that although she knew she should be happy, she wasn't, especially when, as a couple, they were invited to social functions, charity dinners, where she met people who she believed were insincere. We talked of how she felt at these occasions. In response she winced.

'They are so sure of themselves, confident. Full of news about what they are doing, where they are going. I feel I've nothing to talk about with them, I'm not interesting at all. I'm Nigel's wife and the children are away at school.

'You were very unkind to my receptionist; why was that? I asked.

'Did she offend you?'

'Not really, she just seemed so confident, as though she was looking down on me because I need to be here.'

I asked her to think about what she was saying. Could she be sure that what she presumed was the case, was actually what had happened?

We sat in silence for a while, until she admitted in a soft voice 'I'm being nasty to everyone. That's why I'm here. My husband heard you speak at a conference in London. He begged me to come.'

During the next few sessions, Jennie began to understand how easy it is to create our very own giants who we then invite to live in our land of 'milk and honey.' When we do this, it's often because we lose faith in ourselves. Confidence is essential to our sense of well being. Without it we become anxious and may easily believe that other people wish to hurt us, when often this is not the case.

Jennie gained confidence, joined a local writers group and began to take an extra interest in what was happening in the community. We also talked of retraining which she decided to look into. This together with her more positive approach gave her a sense of identity. She had needed a helping hand in order to change her life. She sought guidance, and reassurance as she began to think 'outside the box.'

Many of our own personal 'giants' do not need to frighten us, but we, as individuals, need to know why we see them as we do we can then

Name them,

Claim them,

and throw them away.

If we are lucky enough to find happiness why spoil it by creating giants?

Have courage and remember
        'Courage is Grace under pressure'
to quote Ernest Hemmingway.

'Well I Never!'

'Your naked body should only belong to those who fall in love with your naked soul.'

Charles Chaplin

The Neil Diamond track playing in my car was one of my favourites so I couldn't be blamed for singing along as I sat waiting for my grandson. I had parked close to the house where he was spending time with a friend. Looking at my watch I realized that it would be a twenty five minutes before he was ready to be collected. I had set off early as, being unfamiliar with the area, I did not want to be late.

'Time to myself' I thought indulgently, just me and Neil singing along together.

I unfastened my seat belt, settled myself more comfortably and closed my eyes. Within minutes a coach pulled in front of me, parked up and then proceeded to discharge its passengers. I presumed that they were returning from an outing organised from the pub across the road.

The all male bus passengers, having alighted, wandered off in various directions; some appeared to be a little out of control, wandering from one side of the pavement to the other, whilst others laughed loudly in an inebriated fashion.

From my vantage point it appeared that the coach was now empty, however the vehicle did not move off. It was a warm day. I opened my window and heard raucous laughter accompanied by loud male conversation although I could not make out the exact words. The driver was talking to the last remaining passenger; the bus was not empty after all, my mistake! Time passed and the coach slowly drew away from the kerb.

It was then that I saw a man standing on the pavement. He looked to be in his fifties, he had long, grey, straggly almost shoulder length hair and a cheery smile on his face.

I gaped as he walked across the road towards the pub car park, laughing loudly to himself. I have to admit that I stared and stared, rather rude of me, you may think, but I have no excuse for my behaviour; you see the man I was looking at was completely naked! He was not wearing a stitch of clothing and proceeded to look on the ground as though he had dropped something. I realized he was trying to find somewhere to sit down; probably sensing that inevitably he would fall down!

The car park surface was covered in rough gravel. I hoped he would not sit on that surface. He was holding a mobile phone. It was obvious that he was very drunk and that possibly his companions had played a rather cruel joke on him.

Could he be a prospective bridegroom?

Had this been a daytime stag party? I could only speculate.

I wondered if I should go across and ask if he needed help. Provide something to cover him; the only blanket I carried in the car was the one my dog used when she travelled with me and it was full of dog hairs.

No, I thought, that would be an insult.

Should I go over to him, again I asked myself?

I was still trying to work out if there was anything I could do when a car drove onto the car park. The man on seeing the car staggered towards the back fence.

The car stopped a few yards from him and a very large lady got out. She was in full 'flight' as she shouted very loudly to the man.

'You stupid man, you have let them do it again. Will you never learn? That is the last time you go on an outing with that group of idiots!'

With that, and making no attempt to cover him the woman grabbed hold of his hair and dragged him to the car. She then manhandled him into the front passenger seat, at the same time continuing to lambast him regarding his behaviour. I noted with amazement that she made no attempt whatsoever to cover his naked body.

She drove off the car park; the wheels skidded, causing a shower of gravel to fly into the air.

Sitting in my car I suddenly realized that the scene around me had become so animatedly interesting that poor Neil Diamond had been forgotten. I think I must have been in shock as I turned my CD off, wishing to gather my thoughts and establish that yes, on a warm sunny afternoon I had seen a totally naked man in a very public place.

The door of a nearby house opened; out came my grandson.

'Hi Grandma' he said 'have you been waiting long?'

When we got back to his house and I described what I had seen, eyebrows were raised prior to a lot of hearty laughter, accompanied by the comment 'It could only happen to you,

'Mum, what are you like? ' The laughter continued throughout the afternoon.

I have passed the pub many times since and I have to admit I always smile remembering that poor stark naked gent!

When I related this happening to an audience, I was asked if I was embarrassed. I replied perhaps this feeling would have been experienced by the man had he not been so drunk.

One lady asked if I felt afraid, did I want to drive away? The thought never occurred to me, I had a lovely grandson to collect and one has to keep life in proportion and get priorities right. However it is not a sight that I would want to see again………….. his hair was very unkempt!!

Love's Young Dream

He gave me a long lingering look, and I melted! At sixteen, melting when looked at, long and lingeringly, by the love of my life, was an amazing experience. I felt as though I had entered another world and that as a consequence I knew what true love really felt like. Ours was a chaste love. How could it be otherwise? We both came from strong Roman Catholic families.

Later, when talking with my friend Pat, we were of the opinion that it was enough simply to be near the loves of our respective lives, and to be very careful how we behaved. We had a friend whose older sister, when discovered to be pregnant, had insisted that she and her boyfriend had only ever kissed and we the totally uninformed were none the wiser!

Whilst attending a retreat, a priest who had recently returned from the overseas missions had taken me to one side. 'You should consider the contemplative life, child' he said. 'Think seriously about becoming a bride of Christ.' 'Learn to be sinless and pure.'

When I did not reply, he attempted to make the prospect more attractive by describing the good I could do by working in a leper colony.

I felt sorry for those suffering from this terrible disease but his words frightened me. I will never be a nun I vowed, never ever!

My boyfriends name was Gerard. He was really clever. His school was staffed by Jesuits, the regime hard, and unforgiving. God help any boy who was a dullard in the care of these hostile, controlling men. The nuns who taught at my grammar school were often unpleasant but my life in their care was a lot easier than his.

Gerard was introduced to me by a boy who lived in our road. Frank. Forever in trouble was Frank, with his high spirits and a hatred of the Jesuits. However he did not let the constant corporal punishment change his views. I liked Frank and wished he was my brother.

Gerard and I would meet in Heaton Park; sometimes he would read poems to me and I, in turn, read the verses that I had written. We both shared a love of World War One poets, who wrote with such insight, with such feverish pain of the suffering and futility of war. I already believed myself to be a confirmed pacifist and dreamt of world peace.

He read with such feeling that I was often moved to tears, and I thought that one day he would be a great actor, appearing on the stage at the Palace Theatre in Manchester…'or you could be in a black and white films' I would tell him 'one day you will be famous' I fully believed that this not only could, but would be the case and I would be forever by his side!

Neither of us had any money. We both had Saturday jobs, but in common with each other, we were expected to hand over our meagre earnings to our elders. Gerard's father had been killed in the war, a pilot, shot to smithereens was how Gerard described it. His mother, struggled, and needed every penny that her son earned. Unlike some widows in her position, she had not insisted that he leave school to bring home a wage, but had made sure that his education continued. She wanted him to have a good professional career and to this end she worked long shifts in a local factory.

My mother did not work, however my father was one of the 'bosses' in the steel mill so I felt quite put out that my money was taken almost without comment.

One Friday evening, around six thirty, a warm summer evening, Gerard met me at our usual meeting place, a particular oak tree. As usual he had walked four miles and I roughly about the same distance as we lived in different directions from the city centre.

'I've got some money' he said, and before I could give any response at all, he blurted out 'My mam gave me the milk money to pay him when he comes tonight; she's at work on nights this week, but I think we should use the money for the pictures. We never go anywhere but the park.'

We sat for a while.

'I'm not sure' I said, 'I can't stay out that long, and what about the milkman?' And then for some random, inane reason I asked

'Has he any children?

What if he doesn't collect much tonight ?

….oh Gerard ?'

It was then he cried. I watched as the tears ran down his face. He drew the back of his hand across his cheeks, as though to stop the flow, but his tears did not stop.

I gave him my hanky, clean, well washed and ironed by my diligent mother, and as he scrubbed at his eyes he turned from me.

'I've broken one of the commandments. It's a mortal sin. My mum will be so angry with me, I've let her down. I just wanted to take you somewhere nice.' I put my arms around him and I cried too. We were both aware that we could not use the money it would be sinful and Gerard would have to confess to the priest in the confessional what he had done.

I had my doubts about the sanctity of the confessional, and although I had read about priests who had sacrificed their lives rather than divulge what they heard, I was not sure that was always the case. As Gerard and I sat thinking about sin and its repercussions I realised that he had to get back home as quickly as possible, in time to pay the milkman.

How chaste we were!

How fearful!

But we were young, inexperienced, learning about life, having been given scant guidance or information as to its reality.

Gerard arrived home in time to meet the milkman as he was collecting further down the street.

'Hello, lad' he said as Gerard gave him the money.

'I thought it was strange that your mam hadn't left it for me, she never fails, your mam, never. Not like some folk round 'ere'.

My house had a lovely garden back and front with a field beyond. Gerard lived in a tiny terrace with a back yard, situated in a jumble of streets that marched in straight lines from the main road into the city centre.

Gerard's eyes were brown, like my father's, and indeed

my own. I have always felt that the eyes are the windows to the soul, and the fact that his eyes were brown meant a lot to me, as I had read somewhere that brown eyes indicated kindness and a soft heart.

At sixteen I felt it quite inappropriate to go out with boys who had blue eyes, as I believed I needed kindness and love. I really thought that one day Gerard would ask me to marry him. After all he was two years my senior and we loved to be together.

During the months that followed, we became more fond of each other. I longed for every meeting: thoughts of Gerard filled the days when seeing each other was impossible to arrange. On those days I dreamt of us being married, sitting eating at a long table, our children seated at each side. There would be four of them. Whilst we were seated Gerard and me would read poetry and great literary works to them. So naive was I that I thought that all of this could be arranged if we both prayed hard enough. The God of our religion would smile on us. As time passed I became more and more certain, my love for Gerard was boundless and all consuming as was his love for me..

Winter came and it was cold and dark by early evening. This meant that I was not allowed out. We could only meet on a Saturday afternoon. How long those days between our trysts seem to be; time dragged its feet but I did not lose heart because I knew that Gerard loved me.

Almost a year after the incident with the milk money we met as usual at 'our' tree.

He looked excited, almost joyful as though he was

bursting to tell me something!

'What is it?' I said, although I had already guessed.

My heart fluttered.

We were now able to meet three times a week, and I was sure that, like me, he lived for those precious times spent in each other's company.

I knew what he was about to say.

I knew where my future lay.

I knew, that when he asked me to marry him I would say YES……..! I knew, I was so sure!

The sun was still warm at four o'clock, easily seen in all its glory, beyond the trees. We sat together in the grass and watched. He put his arm around me.

'Are you ready?' he said.

'Ready for my news?'

I knew what he was going to say, and my answer would be yes.

I could already see the two of us at Mass on Sundays, with our brood of children.

Oh how I loved this kind and caring human being!

He tilted my chin towards his face and kissed me. 'Oh Gerard, I love you' - the words remained unspoken in my head as my heart somersaulted

'I've something really important to tell you.'

I closed my eyes and waited, ready to be kissed again.

'I'm going to be a priest' he said.

I opened my eyes…….

'It's all down to you' he continued

'You've helped me to think differently about life, everything in fact.'

I turned away as he went on 'As a priest I can bring about change. I can help so many people and bring them to Christ.'
He went on speaking but I no longer heard his words

The sunlight was gone from the sky and I felt icy cold.
I watched his mouth. He was now talking quickly in an animated way only the odd word pierced my numbness I realized that his dreams stretched far out into the future –and I was not part of those dreams
Suddenly he was kneeling; he tugged at my shoulders pulling me sharply towards him until we both knelt face to face!
'Just think, Vera, if I hadn't met you this would never have happened! I feel at one with God! I'm to be a Jesuit!'

My erstwhile suitor walked me part of the way home, just as he had always done, but this time we did not chat and laugh and talk about the happenings of our uncomplicated lives. Instead he talked not 'to' me but 'at' me; all the time obviously completely oblivious to my pain and disappointment. At last, we came to the place where we had to go our separate ways.
He held me close and gently explained that he already had a place in a Seminary and that he would write and let me know how he was getting on.
'You look so sad.
Wish me luck sweetheart.
I'll make the world a better place,…for you, and for HIM of course!'

He bent towards me, his lips floated past my own and then he took a few steps away only to turn around saying 'I've just thought - I won't be allowed to keep in touch with you. We're not related and the monks are very strict. Never mind, Vera, when I am the Pope's right hand man I will get in touch with you. I imagine I will have enough "clout" then, more freedom to make contact…that's if they don't send me out as a missionary!'

With that he laughed and I saw the absolute joy in his face. It was all-enveloping as though he was consumed with longing but not for me. To him his dreams for the future were real and he was already a part of them. In that moment I knew for the first time in my young life what the word vocation truly meant!

It took time, a long time, for me to forgive: not to forgive Gerard, but to forgive God and all the monks and priests in the whole of the Holy Roman Church.
I had not known that I was in competition with anyone.
I believed we were in love with each other. It would have been bad enough if he loved another girl, but to discover that I was in competition with such a formidable adversary was completely and utterly overwhelming.
After all, I was a mere girl and I could not compete with HIM!
Decades later I heard that Gerard had as he himself predicted risen to rather dizzy heights in the church. This did not come as a surprise to me, as after all I am a woman of discerning taste!

I'll Have You Know...

I couldn't decide what was happening to the elderly gentleman. Before leaving the very large, busy retail outlet customers were waiting in a long queue to pay for their goods. It was the first day of the sale. Prices, already reduced previously, were again cut at the cash desk by a further ten percent, but only for a limited period. The place was full of life as shoppers moved, at speed, in an attempt to secure a bargain. Although it was merely mid-September Christmas had come early to this outlet, and it was sometimes difficult to avoid shopping trolleys carrying bulky, festive merchandise.

As I approached the cash point with its huge sign, requesting 'Pay Here', I wondered how long I would have to wait in order to do precisely that and escape!

It was then I caught sight of the elderly man, as he stooped, and appeared to be losing his balance. There was a long gap between him and the next trolley pusher. He did not have a trolley. As I approached, he began to fall further forward..

'Are you alright?' I enquired.

He did not look up as he was trying to regain his balance One of his walking sticks fell to the floor.

I bent down, picked it up and handed it to him.

He looked at me with grey, rheumy eyes.

I repeated myself.

'Are you alright?'

'Can I help you?

'I'm trying to fasten my jacket button.' He said.

'Would you like me to fasten it for you?'

Although it was obvious that his body was well stooped, possibly due to age, he attempted to raise his head and looked straight at me.

It was then I sensed the anger. However, nothing could have prepared me for his next words…

'I'll have you know madam that I'm a happily married man', he declared in a loud angry voice.

So loud in fact that several people waiting in the queue looked at him, and then frowning, looked questioningly at me.

I waited for a smile, any small, slight indication that his words were said in jest, but all I sensed was his almost uncontrollable rage.

My mind raced, perhaps he was cross because he was very independent and resented being offered help, but I sensed it was more than that.

Then with his walking stick, the very stick that had previously fallen to the floor, which I had bent to pick up, he pointed towards a woman standing ahead of us, waiting in the queue with her heavily laden trolley.

He shouted 'And that's my wife over there and she can see what you are doing to me. We are happily married!'

The aforementioned woman was glaring at me so much that I was momentarily rendered speechless. What had I done other than offer to help some one?

If only they knew what an effort it had been for me to offer to pick up the walking stick in the first place.

It's safe to say that, as I bent down to do so, I did

wonder if I would be able to straighten up myself, as I'm not getting any younger, and bending is sometimes a problem.

However, I did manage to respond to the man's outburst with a gallows laugh, accompanied with the retort 'How ridiculous....... chance would be a fine thing!'

With this said, I turned my back on the unpleasant gent, only for his wife to continue to glare at me from further along the line for what seemed an age as the automated voice continued to let us know which cashier was available. However the wife, undaunted by the opposition, shouted to her husband asking him if he was alright. By which time several people waiting in the queue were staring at me.

Later, when I returned to the car, I sat for quite a time. That will teach me, I thought, not to offer help but I reasoned it would be a problem to me, if I did *not* offer help

I believe, that if we show each other kindness, we will help counteract the badness in the world.

Being kind to others usually has a positive effect.

It puts a deposit in the recipient's 'Emotional Bank'.

It also places a deposit, emotionally, with the giver.

If everyone showed kindness to each other we would lead more positive lives. I'm not suggesting that 'good deeds' stop wars and conflict, but I do believe if we want to be at peace with our own inner selves, we have to appreciate that we have to start by making a set of choices as to how we lead our lives. We have to look outside ourselves, rather than constantly looking in!

As I continued to sit in the car, windows open,

The sun shining,

A gentle breeze wafting through,

I felt so grateful for life itself.

Then my thoughts returned to my recent experience.

I wondered what kind of a man I had encountered.

With my professional experience I believe he was not suffering from dementia. His face, though aged, carried faded evidence of how handsome he must once have been. Maybe a 'ladies man' in his era, who had chosen to marry a plain-featured girl, whose own face, now decades later, showed believable evidence of her life long aptitude for scowling and sulking!

Did they still love each other?

They obviously had a family, or so the Christmas themed contents of their shopping trolley would suggest, but why his outburst?

Did he think that he was being propositioned by me?

That I wanted to run off with him into the sunset?

How ludicrous,

How very hilarious….can you imagine?

And as I sat, I began to laugh.

Not a small laugh.

I wanted to laugh from deep down inside.

There are some days when it is so wonderful to be alive.

And yet there would be those shoppers passing by, who,

seeing a smart, yet elderly woman, laughing loudly, sitting alone in her four by four might think

'How very odd.'

But you can depend on the fact that they would quicken their steps to get away from such behaviour, for sadly, so many of us are programmed from an early age not to get involved, not even to appear to notice what is happening around us.

To leave the car park, I had to take a round about route due to the one-way system. It was then, whilst involved in such a detour, that I saw him in the distance.

A slowly walking stooped man.

Wearing a straw hat

Aided by the use of two sticks,

Jacket flapping in the breeze

Possibly due to the fact that none of his buttons were fastened!

Suddenly, it was as though we were the only two people at this end of the car park.

What was he doing down here?

Then I saw what was presumably his car, well, *their* car, parked so far away from the main entrance, albeit beside a trolley park!

I had to stop as he walked in front of me.

I doubt he was aware of my presence, or indeed of any approaching vehicle.

Little did he know that I had, and still have, a further message for him.

Old man, I want you to know you did not embarrass me with your behaviour. In fact you actually made my day. Prior to meeting you, I had no notion that I am, obviously, in fact a mature 'femme fatale', and you must really have a high opinion of yourself, or perhaps you are ageing in anger, longing for the days when you were young.

After my encounter with you,

I smiled as I drove along the motorway,

I smiled as I meandered thoughtfully through the little picturesque villages close to my home.

And I was still laughing and smiling as I talked later on the telephone to a close friend who lives at the other end of the country.

My dear old gent - what joy meeting you has brought me!

Thank you.

You made a big deposit in my emotional bank. However, on this occasion, no return deposit went into yours. You see, to use the emotional banking system, one has to be aware of how precious this life really is!

WE really need to be aware!

Not a Prayer...
Just a Chat

When am I going to die Lord?

When will I hear the call?

Will it be loud as a trumpet or hardly a whisper at all?

Will you give me some warning so that I can prepare?

Or will it be all of a sudden before I am simply not there?

I say I'm not frightened of dying that my faith in you is so strong but really I fear that I'm lying and often I think Lord how long?

My thoughts are not morbid or heavy it's simply this worry I have that I won't be fully prepared Lord and I think that would make me feel bad.

Lord really I know that you love me I so want to trust in your care but deep down inside I am fearful that when the time comes you're not there.

I won't mind dying in sunshine, a spring day is probably best, but please don't take me at twilight my spirit would never quite rest.

My dad hated dusk, that space between daylight and night he said it's not one or the other and that it could never feel right.

When I was young I imagined a deathbed scene was the best, lots of sighing instructions, weeping, wailing and rest.

But as the years passed all that changed and common sense moved in, a priest would be more important on account of all my sin.

Lord I do hope you're listening although this isn't a prayer cos I really need you, you know that. I've got to believe that you're there.

Oh Lord there's just one more detail I nearly forgot to include on the day when I'm turned into ashes when my family feel lost and in grief would you please send a rainbow to cheer them it would bring them such blessed relief!

Vera Waters

Another Thought

On several occasions during my working life, I have been approached by journalists, who have asked if they could write my biography. I have always refused feeling that this was something I did not want to do. I believed it to be an intrusion into my private life and the lives of my very precious family.. However, when reviewing this, my sixth book, I realise that so much of it is, in fact, autobiographical. This was *not* my intention when I began to formulate the content.

I am very fortunate in that my life has been full of opportunity and the sound of doors opening. When I became aware that this was happening I decided to step through those portals believing that in so doing I would find new, exciting experiences. Rarely have I hesitated and the result has been that my career has proved to be very interesting and varied.

You may or may not believe in *serendipity - the gift of making fortunate discoveries by accident,* I must say that I do believe because so often there is no logical explanation for things that happen to us.

Sometimes people ask me how I have managed to do so much. It is then that I point out that my career has already spanned over fifty years and hopefully continues! However it was necessary for me to leave the security of the N.H.S. to branch out into the private sector. It was a big step but again I believed another door would open.

I was correct in my assumption I became the first counsellor to be retained by two police forces and was awarded a research grant from the home office, the only civilian to do so at that time. It was very special to me as the award came from the department of science & technology and of course counselling is not considered to be scientific in any way . During that period of my life I trained police officers from twenty one forces.

An interesting door opened for me when I met the Welfare Officer from the Northern Lighthouse Board. As a result of this meeting I was invited to visit several of the Scottish Lighthouses prior to automation. I met such amazing men from whom I learned of the history of this noble profession. Later I met some of their wives who gave me memorable insights into their unique way of life.

When a major airline requested to retain me as a Trainer and Counsellor, I was pleased to accept but was not to know that this would involve my training their staff in Berlin, a very interesting door had opened due to my meeting a man named Michael , who has remained a friend ever since.

Within months of that experience, I was invited to visit Perth, Australia, having been unexpectedly, although not literally, catapulted to the other side of the world, a further door had definitely opened enabling me to present at a senior police chief's symposium and to be interviewed on the radio. This happened as a direct result of a sad event in my life which made me feel that an adventure might be part of the healing process!

For me serendipity is a fact of life; for instance, my work in America came about because on one summer's day I boarded a train to Edinburgh. Whilst travelling on that train I met a lady who lived in Virginia. The train was delayed and as a consequence we both missed our connection to Perth thus we spent several hours in each others company.

As we chatted, she invited me to visit her. Although I had never previously considered flying across the pond it was completely without hesitation that I agreed. The result was that within months, I was sitting enjoying a cup of tea in her lounge. She and her husband introduced me to other interesting people. The lady on the train was Phyllis she is married to Joe we are still close friends

This led to me being asked to provide training for various professional groups throughout Virginia and the surrounding states due to the help of a man named Rick. And yes we are still in touch. When he arranged for me to speak in Chicago yet another door had opened!

Happily I returned to that amazing city to speak on several more occasions! It was at that first presentation I met Scott Lebin who has written the introduction at the beginning of this book.

There is so much I could say here, including meeting a lady on a westbound Trans-Atlantic crossing. We began our conversation by her admiring the piece of patchwork I was sewing at the time. Much later this conversation led to my being invited to train members of the Governors departmental staff in Oklahoma. The theme being 'Self Awareness & Management Skills', that sea traveller was Betty later I met her husband John, again we remain friends.

More recently, I felt honoured to be presented to The Princess Royal as a result of being commissioned by 'Bookbite' to write articles that would encourage older people to feel more positive about their lives.

The doors, thankfully, continue to open, although now, I hear my mouth make promises that my body can no longer keep! However it's wonderful to be in a position to choose exactly what I want to do, but believe me, if a very interesting door opens, I will be through it in a trice with a smile on my face !

Despite everything I've written here it is important to remember that we are all human and to 'err is human.'

Blind confidence is not attractive, to have some humility is important if we are to retain our friendships and truly influence the lives of others.

We are not always right nor do we have all the answers there is so much we can learn from each other.

During my first teaching practice many years back a wonderful wise headmaster in a primary school taught me the most important lesson of my life..
I was entering a classroom when he bade me wait a moment to consider what he was about to say
'Miss, remember the children you are to teach may know far more about life than you'
Audaciously but with some temerity I ventured to say
'They are only four years old '
'precisely' was his response
'That is exactly the point I am making.'

I have never forgotten and whenever I speak to groups I remind myself of his words; of course some of the members of my audiences will be much more erudite and more clever than me!
But when I speak I am the one 'daring greatly' in the arena as Roosevelt said.

Our lives are full of interaction from the very simple to the complex. Leave yourself open to serendipity everything happens for a purpose perhaps that is why you are reading these words!

Another door opening for you!!!!!!!!

The 'After…words.'

I am surrounded by paper, some of which is covered with printed words, tangible proof that my thoughts and ideas eventually were transferred to my desk top computer that boasts two screens! But then there is a veritable mountain of paper, covered in my pencilled hand writing. If proofed in green ink, it is ready, either to find its way into my next book, or be sent, when typed, as an article to a journal of my choice. The hungry teeth of the shredder look inviting, and as the book is now complete, the process of sorting and tidying up begins. My work place, to a passing stranger might, or on second thoughts, definitely appear to be a chaotic shambles, but to me it is a place of comfort and growth; a haven where my ideas take formal shape; a place where my thoughts become words and stories.

We are all story tellers, for every life is a story, a real story, totally unique to you as the teller, because no two people have identical experiences. Our lives are important. The contribution that each of us make to the wholeness of our short existence on this planet is incredibly precious, and needs to be acknowledged and valued accordingly. We do not exist in isolation, and it is because of this fact that we can, if we wish, affect the lives of so many people. The choice is ours as to whether that interaction is positive or negative.

I hope that, whilst reading, you have experienced varied emotions, and at some point found yourself thinking 'I do that' or 'Why did that happen?' My aim was to give you food for thought and in so doing reach into your heart! Until we meet again, may your god go with you.

Thank you.
Vera Waters, Summer 2017

Also available

RAINBOW CONNECTIONS
True Reflections
2012, ISBN 9780951695258
A further collection of inspirational true stories
presented in the author's familiar style. As in her
previous books, humour and pathos prevail together
with common sense, advice and insight.

Also an ebook for Amazon Kindle and in Apple iTunes

STRONG TEA & BISCUITS
True tales to encourage & inspire
2007, ISBN 9780951695241

RECIPE FOR A RAINBOW
Inspirational Stories of Everyday Life
2004, ISBN 0951695223

THE OTHER HALF OF THE RAINBOW
True Stories and Inspirational Advice
1996, ISBN 0951695215

HALF A RAINBOW
Insight Into Stress
1990, reprinted 1997, ISBN 0951695207

CDs   LITTLE BY LITTLE
WHERE DO YOU KEEP THE GUITAR

Dedications and signed copies available. To book Vera for talks, presentations, lectures or coaching and to purchase any of the above.

www.verawaters.com

Tel 0845 8387403

Or write to,
Penn Cottage Books
PO Box 121
Chorley
Lancashire
PR6 8GF
UK

Books also available at discerning bookshops.

Follow Vera on Twitter @vera_waters

'Angels fly because
they take themselves lightly'

G. K. Chesterton